Skeletal
&
Muscular Systems

Concise
Bulleted
Lecture Notes

By
Mostafa ElNaggar

Part 2/7
Human A&P Booklet
with Clinical Implications

ISBN

***

Skeletal
&
Muscular Systems

Concise
Bulleted
Lecture Notes

By
Mostafa ElNaggar

Part 2/7
Human A&P Booklet
with Clinical Implications

ISBN

Contents

Preface

- This **concise** booklet offers the basic anatomical & physiological framework with clinical applications.
- It gives the **direct information** required to understand the subject and pass the test.
- It includes all the important information, in a **bulleted** form, with **simple language** and straight forward presentation.
- It is supported with **figures** and **diagrams** to clarify the important concepts.
- It allows you to study in small digestible bits of information, instead of using large, **boring textbook.**
- It is useful when teaching is in an **integrated** curriculum.
- You can go through it **very quickly**, and use it as a **quick revision** before the examination.
- You can select to read the material **relevant** to you and review it **several times** until you master it.
- It follows the standard **learning outcomes**.
- It could be supported with any **Atlas** of anatomy.
- It is designed to be taught in **one or two courses** of 3-6 credit hours.
- The booklet is published as one part or divided into **7 parts** to make it suitable for e-publishing.

Chapter 3: Skeletal system

A & P of bones *(Repeated from Chapter 1)*

Functions of the bones

1. **Support** the body
2. **Protect** certain structures (eg brain, spinal cord, heart, lungs)
3. Provide **attachment** for skeletal muscles
4. Provide storage for **minerals**: as calcium, phosphate
5. Formation of **Blood elements**: in red marrow
6. Storage of **fat**: in yellow marrow
7. Production of **hormone**: **osteocalcin** (regulates insulin secretion).

Bone markings

- **Projections**: for muscle attachment
  - Tubercle: small projection
  - Tuberosity: large projection
  - Ridge: linear projection
  - Epicondyle: projection over condyle
  - spine
- **Surfaces**: for joints
  - head
  - facet
  - condyle
- **Depressions** & **foramina**: for vessels & nerves
  - groove
  - fissure
  - foramen
  - notch
  - fossa
  - sinus
  - meatus

Structure of the long bone *(Fig. 1)*

- Shaft = **diaphysis**: compact bone, then spongy bone, surrounding marrow cavity
- 2 ends = **epiphysis**: compact & spongy bone, surrounding marrow cavities.
  - covered with hyaline cartilage
- Epiphyseal **line**, between epiphysis & diaphysis
  - is a remnant of **epiphyseal plate** (growth plate)
- **Periosteum**: contain osteoblasts & osteoclasts

- **Endosteum**: lines the marrow cavity

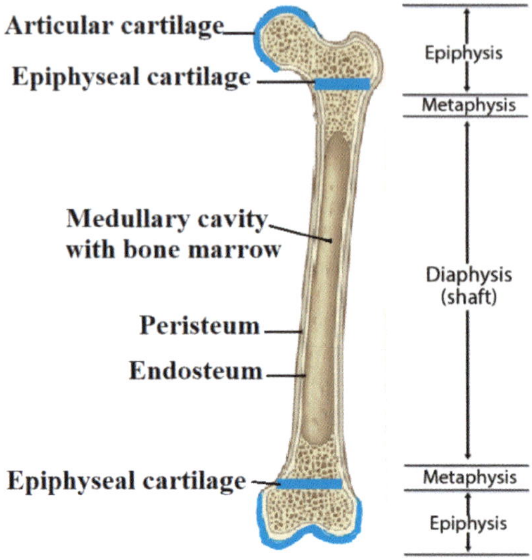

Figure 1: Structure of long bone

<u>**Classification of bones**</u>

According to <u>shape</u>:

- **Long** bones: bones of the limbs, have 2 ends + shaft
- **Short** bones: bones of wrist & ankle
- **Flat** bones: bones of the skull, ribs, sternum, scapula
- **Irregular** bones: vertebrae, hip bone

According to <u>position</u>:

- **Axial** skeleton: skull, vertebrae, ribs
- **Appendicular** skeleton: upper & lower girdles, limbs

According to <u>structure</u>: ***(Figs. 2, 3)***

- **Compact** bone: dense, smooth bone
  - arranged in concentric layers of units called **osteons (Haversian system)**
  - e.g. outer surface of long bones
- **Spongy** bone: trabecular spaces, filled with red or yellow marrow

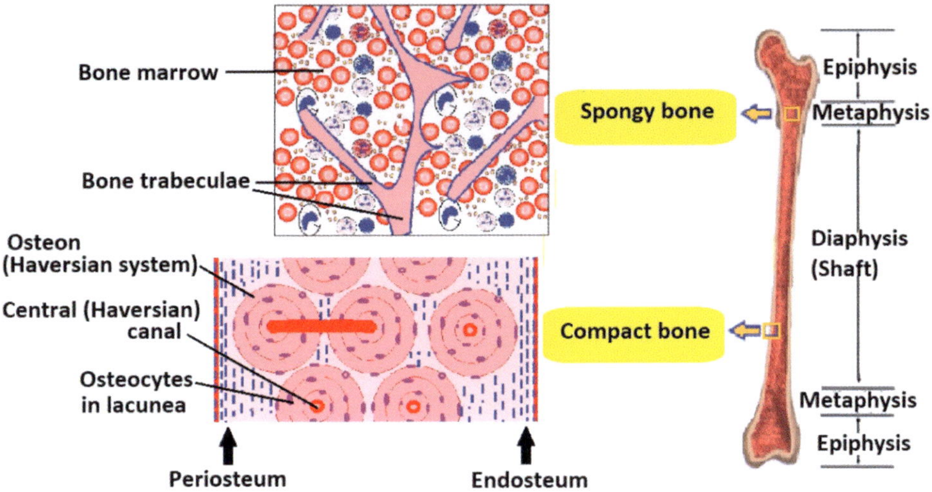

Figure 2: Compact and spongy bones

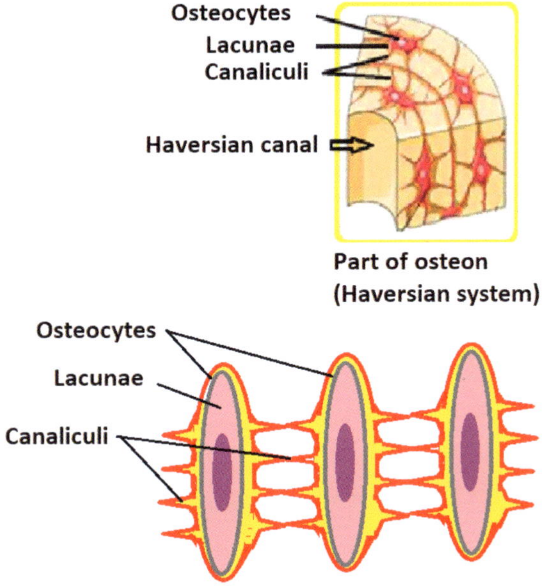

Figure 3: Structure of compact bone

<u>Cells of bone tissue</u> *(Fig. 4)*

- **osteogenic** cells = **osteoprogenitor** cells: active stem cells → divide & give osteoblasts
- **osteoblasts**: → secrete bone matrix (osteoid) →
- **osteocytes**: present inside lacunae and have canaliculi →
  - maintain bone matrix
  - take part in bone remodeling

- **osteoclasts**: have ruffled border
  - →bone resorption

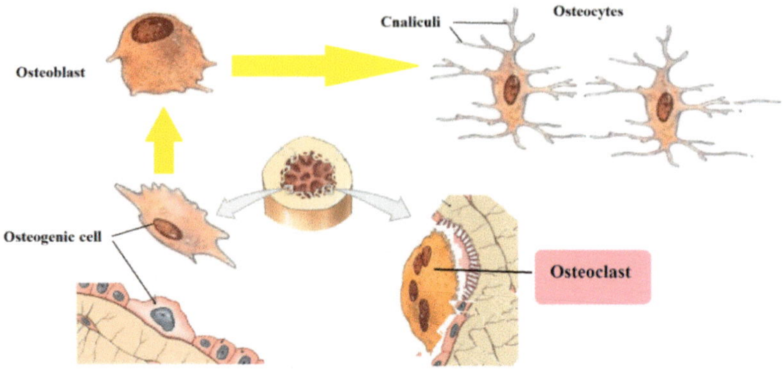

Figure 4: Cells of bone tissue

<u>Bone ossification</u> ***(Fig. 5)***
2 types: endochondral, intramembraneous
Endochondral: bone replaces hyaline cartilage, occur in long bones

- In the **<u>diaphysis:</u>** → gives bone collar + primary ossification center
  - Medullary cavity develops
- In **<u>epiphysis</u>** → gives secondary ossification center
  - Hyaline cartilage remains in
    - Epiphyseal plate: for growth of the bone in length
    - Articular cartilage: for joints
- **Appositional growth (to increase diameter)** occur by bone resorption from the inner surface & bone deposition on the outer surface

Intramembranous: bone develops in fibrous connective tissue
- as in the skull cap (cranium)

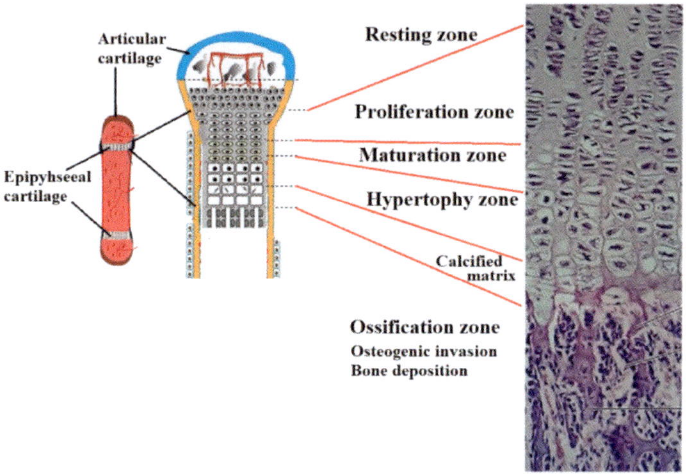

Figure 5: Endochondral ossification

Chemical composition of bone

- **Organic**: cells + osteoid (ground substance + collagen)
- **Inorganic** (65%): hydroxyapatite (calcium phosphate)

Bone disorders

- **Osteomalacia**: poorly mineralized, soft, weak bones
  - treated with calcium & vitamin D
- **Rickets**: the same as osteomalacia, but in children
  - gives bowed legs
- **Osteoporosis**: bone resorption more than bone deposition
  - Occur in menopause women
  - matrix is normal
  - bone mass decline
  - treated by calcium & vitamin D
  - **Causes**: after 65 in males, after menopause (50) in females
  - **Investigation**: dual-energy X-ray absorptiometry **(DEXA)**
  - **Treatment**:
    - **bisphosphonates** → inhibit osteoclast cells
    - **Calcitonin** → inhibit osteoclasts
    - **parathyroid** → stimulates osteoblasts
- **Paget's disease**: excessive abnormal bone resorption and deposition
  - gives deformity

Repair of broken bone

(a) Hematoma forms between the broken parts of the bone →
(b) Fibrocartilage fills the space for 3 weeks →
(c) Osteoblast cells → form **Bony callus** →
(d) Osteoclast cells → reabsorb bone excess→ **Bone remodeling**

Skeleton
The skeleton is divided into
I. Axial skeleton

- skull (cranium & face bones)
- vertebrae
- ribs

II. Appendicular skeleton

- Upper limb
- Lower limb

Axial skeleton

The skull is formed by

- cranium
- facial bones

- It contains **paranasal air sinuses,** which open into the nose.
  - maxillary
  - frontal
  - sphenoidal
  - ethmoidal
- **Sinusitis** = inflammation of the paranasal sinuses.
- **Mastoiditis** = inflammation of mastoid sinuses → leads to deafness.
  - The mastoid sinus drains into the middle ear.

The Skull Cranium: formed of 8 bones (Fig. 6)

- Surround & protect the brain
- Contains **vault** & **base** (its inside is the **cranial cavity**, which has ant, middle & post cranial fossae)

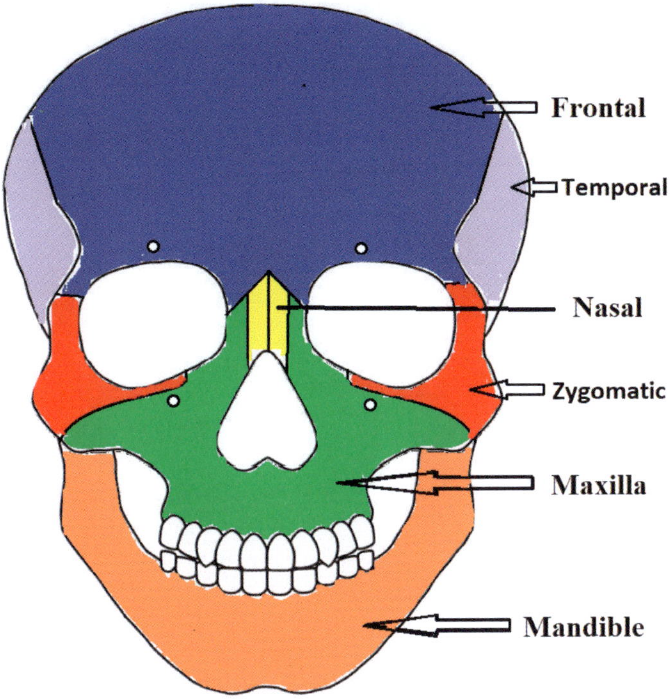

Figure 6: Anterior view of the skull

Skull vault: composed of (Figs. 6 & 7)

- **Bones**:
  - 1 **frontal bone**: forms the superior margin of the orbit
  - 1 **occipital bone**: contains
    - foramen magnum
    - occipital condyles that articulate with the first cervical vertebra (atlas)
  - 2 temporal bones
  - 2 parietal bones
  - 1 sphenoid bone
  - 1 ethmoid bone

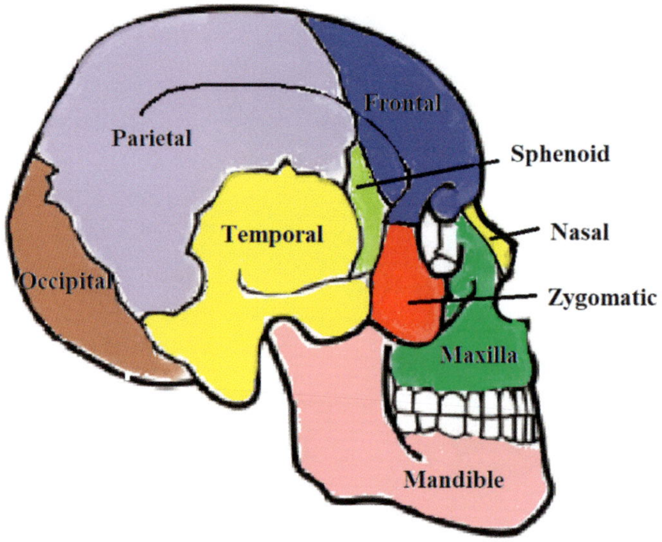

Figure 7: Lateral view of the skull

- **Sutures**: where bones meet (Fig. 8)
  - **Coronal** suture: where parietal meet the frontal
  - **Sagittal** suture: between the 2 parietal bones
  - **Lambdoid** suture: parietal bones meet the occipital
- **Fontanelles** (Fig. 3)
  - Ant fontanelle: closes at 18-24 months
  - Post fontanelles: closes at 6 months

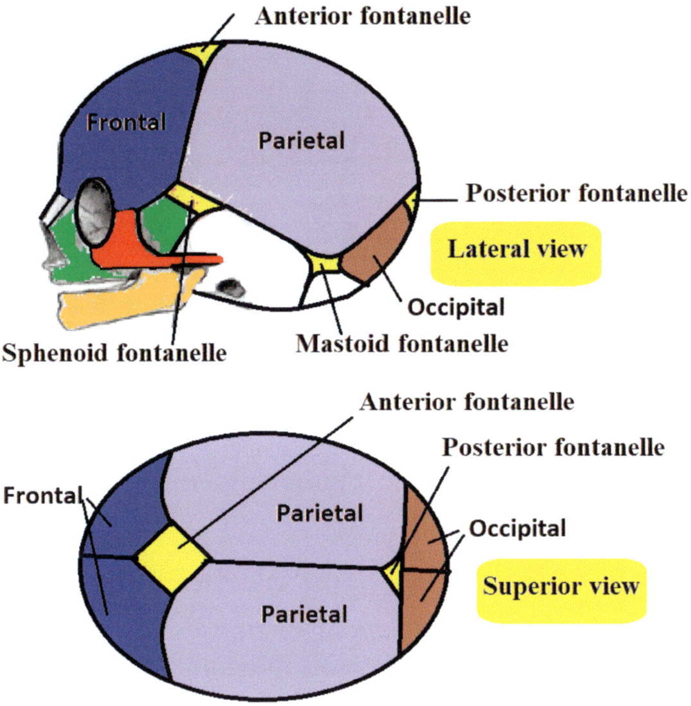

Figure 8: Fontanelles of the fetal skull

<u>**Temporal bone**:</u> has the following features (Fig. 9):

- **Squamous part** of temporal bone
- **external auditory meatus**: is a canal → leads to the middle ear
- **mandibular fossa** → articulates with the mandible
- **mastoid process** → provides attachment for neck muscles
- **styloid process** → provides attachment for muscles of the tongue and larynx
- **zygomatic process** → forms the cheek bone

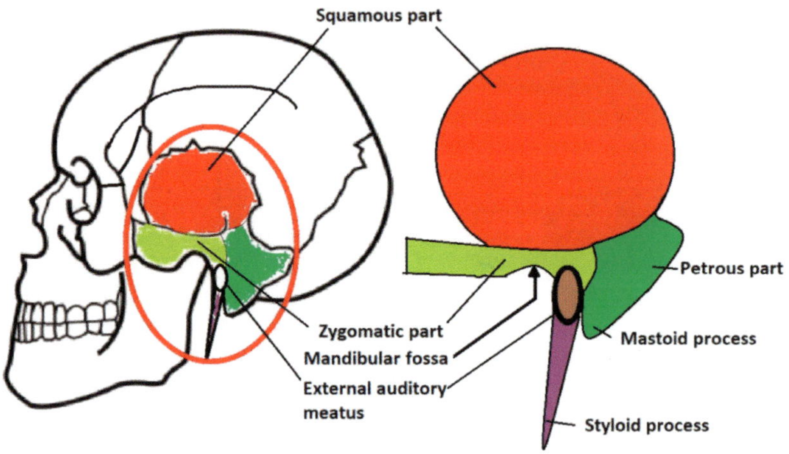

Figure 9: Temporal bone

<u>Sphenoid bone</u>

- ties the cranial bones together
- Components (Figs. 10 & 11)
  - **Body**: contains 2 sphenoid air sinuses, sella turcica, hypophyseal fossa (contains the pituitary gland)
  - **Greater wings**
  - **Lesser wings**
  - **Pterygoid processes**/ plates (medial & lateral)
  - **Foramina**: optic canal, foramen rotundum, foramen ovale, foramen spinosum, super orbital fissure

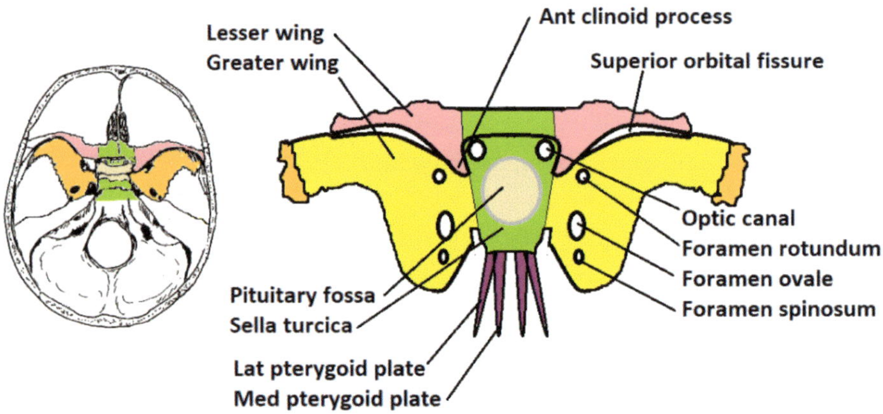

Figure 10: Sphenoid bone

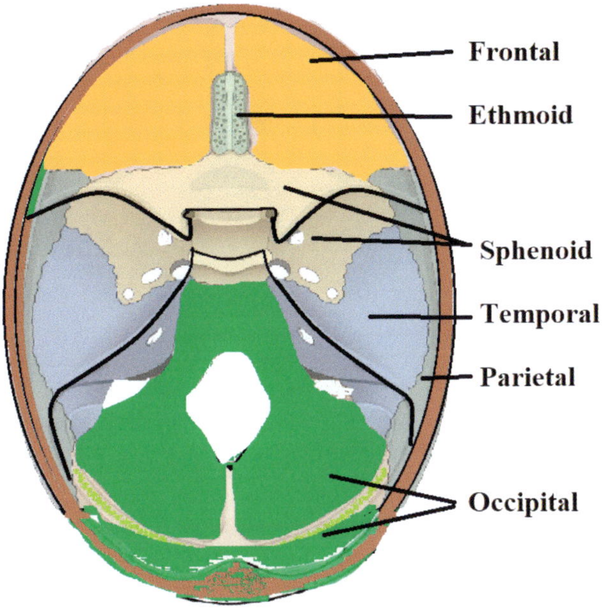

Figure 11: Cranial cavity

Ethmoid bone

- Lies anterior to the sphenoid bone
- Components: (Figs. 11 & 12)
  - **Crista galli**
  - **Cribriform plate**
  - **perpendicular plate** (nasal septum)
  - **Lateral mass**: ethmoidal air cells, **superior & middle conchae**
  - **Orbital plate**

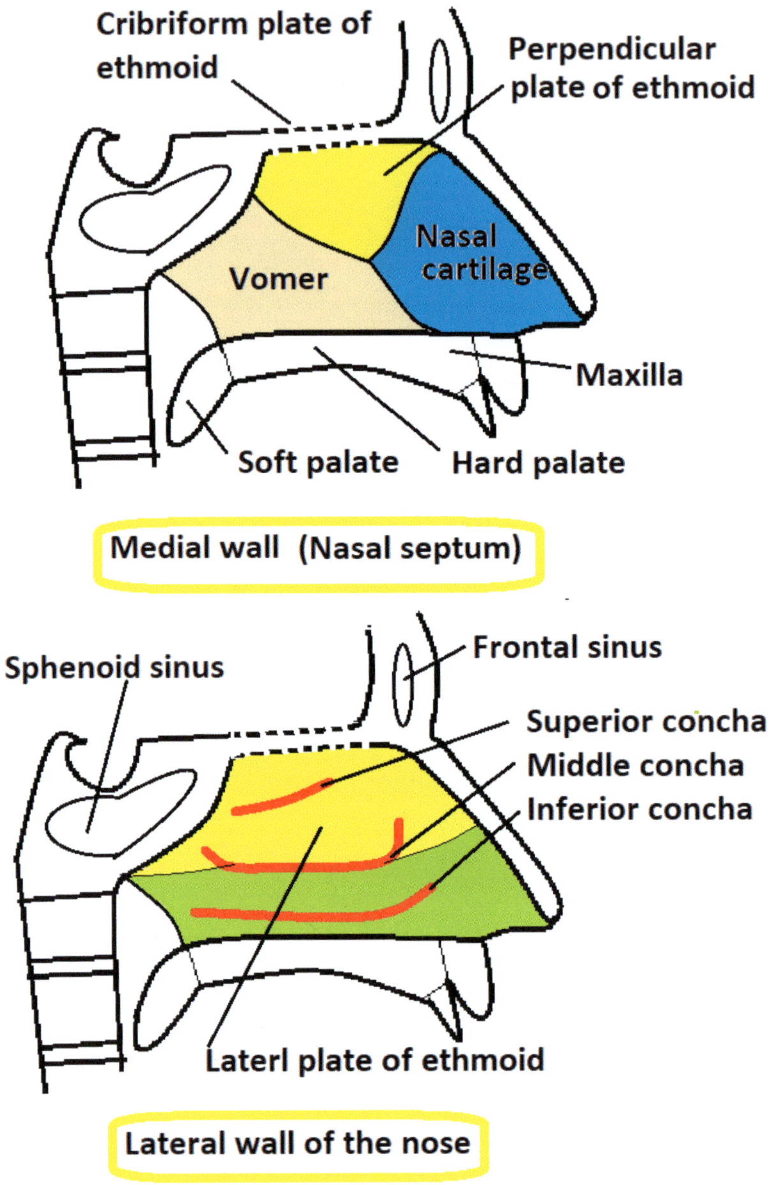

Figure 12: Nasal cavity and ethmoid bone

<u>**Bones of the face**</u> (Figs. 6 & 7)

- Maxilla
- Palatine
- Zygomatic
- Lacrimal
- Nasal
- Vomer

- Mandible

Maxilla

- Components (Fig. 13)
  - **Alveolar process**: forms the sockets of upper teeth
  - **Palatine process**: form the anterior portion of the hard palate (roof of the mouth)
  - Floor of the orbit
  - Sides of the floor of the nasal cavity

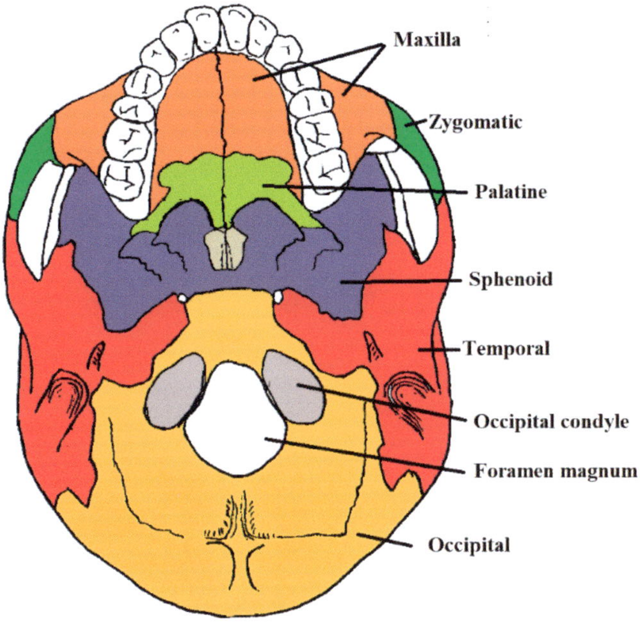

Figure 13: Base of the skull

Palatine bone

- contributes to:
  - Floor and lateral wall of the nasal cavity
  - The **horizontal plates** of the palatine bones (Fig. 8) → form the posterior portion of the **hard palate**
- **Cleft palate**: results from failure of fusion of the 2 horizontal plates of the palatine bones

Zygomatic bone

Components: (Figs. 6 & 7)

- Lateral wall of the orbit
- **Temporal process → Zygomatic arch:** most of the cheek bone

Other small bones

- **Lacrimal Bones:** located on the medial walls of the orbits.
  - **Lacrimal duct**: present between the orbit and the nasal cavity → duct for tears
- **Nasal Bones:** → forms the bridge of the nose.
- **Vomer Bone:** joins with the perpendicular plate of the ethmoid bone → to form the nasal septum (Fig. 12)
- **Inferior Nasal Conchae:** (Fig. 12)
  - at the lateral wall of the nasal cavity. (Note that superior and middle nasal conchae are parts of the ethmoid bone.)

Mandible: Body + 2 rami (Fig. 14)

- **Body**:
  - alveolar process (have the sockets of the lower teeth)
  - mandibular foramen (for inf alveolar N, from V3)
  - mental foramen: for mental nerve
  - **Inferior alveolar canal** between mandibular foramen & mental foramen:
    - contains inferior alveolar N (from V3)
- **Ramus**:
  - mandibular notch
  - 2 processes (coronoid + condylar)

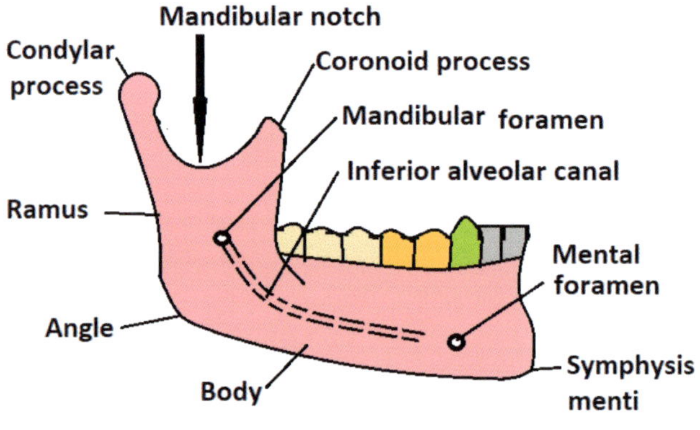

Figure 14: Mandible

Vertebral column

- 33 vertebrae (75%) + intervertebral discs (25%) (Fig. 15)
- **Mnemonics**: their **number** similar to the common meal times: 7 AM, 12 noon, 5 PM
  - Cervical 7
  - Thoracic 12

- Lumbar 5
- Sacral 5
- Coccygeal 3-5

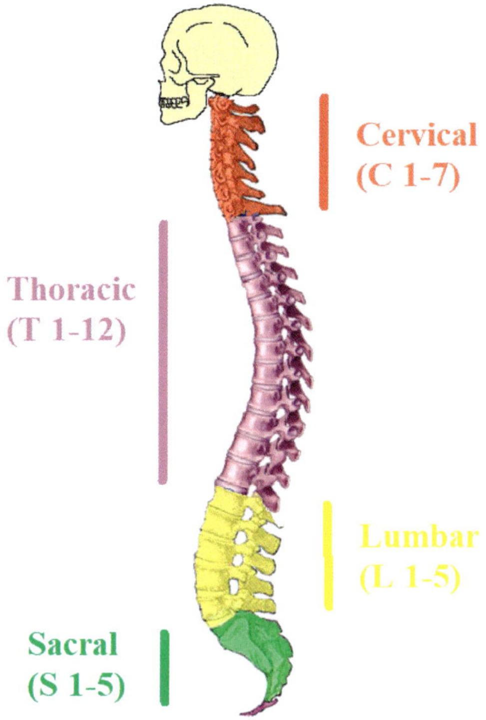

Figure 15: Vertebral column

- S-shaped, with 4 curvatures: (Fig. 15)
  - **cervical** and **lumbar**: convex ant
  - **thoracic** and **sacral**: concave ant

Abnormal curvatures (Fig. 16)

- **Scoliosis**: Lateral thoracic curvature
- **Kyphosis** = **hunchback**: dorsal thoracic curvature
- **Lordosis** = swayback: increased lumbar curvature, due to tuberculosis, osteomalacia or pregnancy

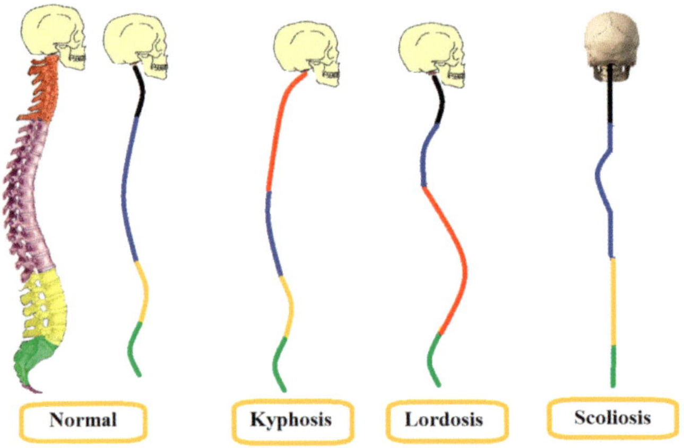

Figure 16: Abnormal curvatures of the vertebral column

Intervertebral disc

- **2 components** (Fig. 17)
  - **Nucleus pulposus**: inner gelatinous
  - **Annulus fibrosus**: outer, fibrocartilage
- Function: Absorb shock during walking, running and jumping
- Herniated **(prolapsed) disc:** due to rupture of the annulus fibrosus → protrusion of the nucleus pulposus → compresses the spinal cord or spinal nerves
  - Treatment
    - 90%: spontaneous cure
    - 5%: surgery as laminectomy, minimally invasive discotomy

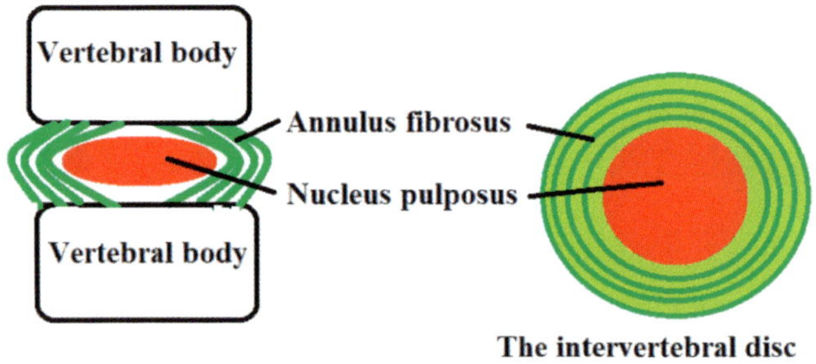

Figure 17: The intervertebral disc

Structure of vertebra (Fig. 18)

- **Body**: connected by intervertebral discs & ligaments

- **Arch**:
  - **Have 2 components**
    - **Pedicle**: intervertebral foramen between 2 pedicles
    - **Lamina** attached by the ligamentum flavum
  - **vertebral foramen** (canal) present between the arch & the body
- **Processes**
  - Spinous process
  - Transverse process
  - Superior articular process
  - Inferior articular process

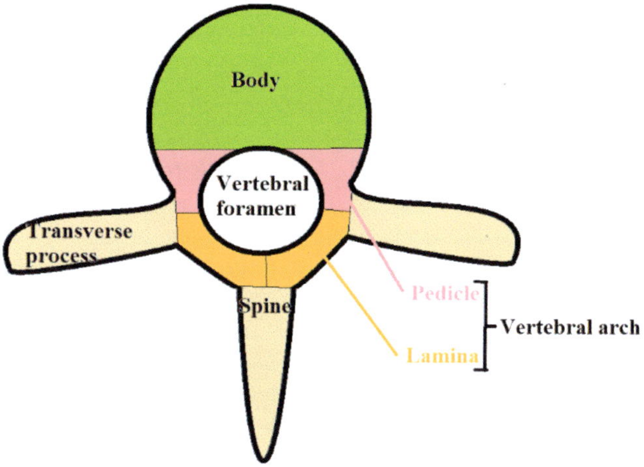

Figure 18: The structure of the vertebra

<u>**Articulation (connection) of two vertebrae**</u>

- Bodies of vertebrae
  - **Intervertebral discs**: cartilaginous joints
  - Ant longitudinal lig
  - Post longitudinal lig
- Sup & inf articular processes: Synovial joints
- Laminae: **Lig flavum**
- Spines: supraspinous & interspinous ligs
- Transverse processes: intertransverse ligs

Specific features of the different vertebrae (Fig. 19)
(key features are colored red)

Feature	**Cervical (3-7)**	**Thoracic**	**Lumbar**
Body	Small, oval	Heart-shaped + **costal facets**	**Large, Kidney-shaped**

Transverse process	**foramen transversarium**	**Costal facets**	Thin
Spinous process	**Short, bifid**	Long, sharp	Short, rectangular
Vertebral foramen	Triangular	Circular	Triangular
Sup. Art. process	Directed sup. Post.	Directed post.	Directed medially
Inf. Art. process	Directed inf. Ant.	Directed ant.	Directed laterally
Movement	Greatest range	Rotation	Flexion & extension

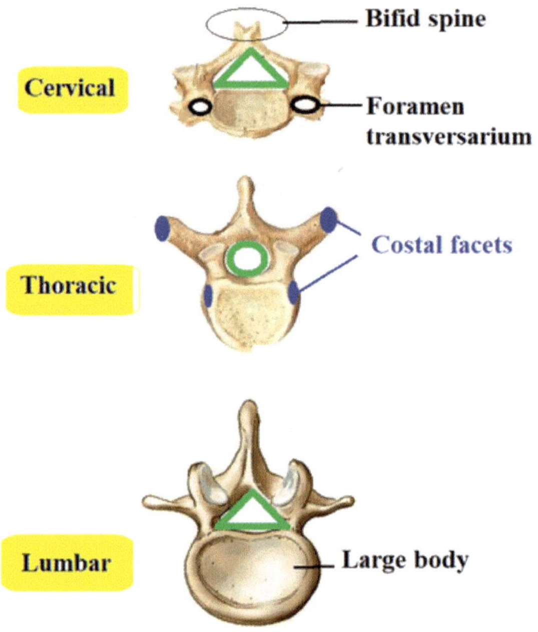

Figure 19: Features of different vertebrae

Special types of vertebrae

Atlas (C1) (Fig. 20)

- No body, no spine
- **Components**
  - **Ant & post arches**
  - 2 **lateral masses**

- **Sup articular process**: articulate with the occipital condyles
- **inf articular process**: articulate with the axis

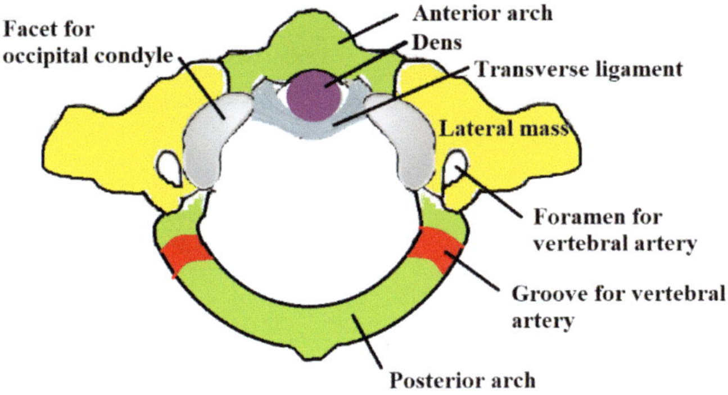

Figure 20: Atlas vertebra

<u>**Axis**</u> **(C2)** (Fig. 21)

- **Dens** (**Odontoid process**) projects upwards from the body

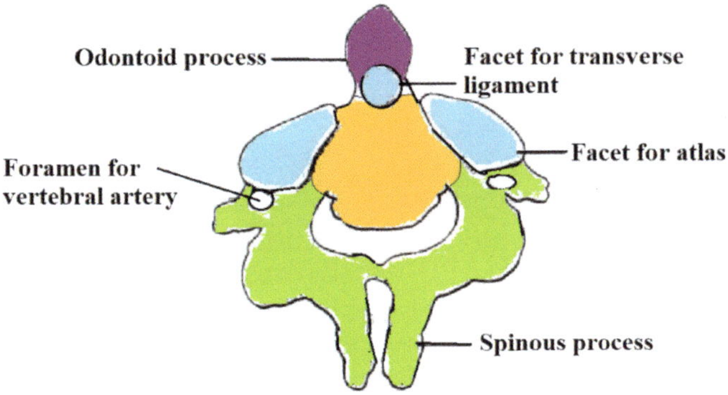

Figure 21: Axis vertebra

<u>**Sacrum**</u>

- Triangular bone (Fig. 22)
- Formed by attachment of 5 sacral vertebrae (S1-S5)
- Vertebral foramina → form **sacral canal**
- Components
  - **Base** (S1): ala of sacrum, sacral promontory
  - **Ant surface**: 4 transverse ridges & 4 ant sacral foramina (for ant rami of sacral Ns)
  - **Post surface**: median (fused spines) & lateral sacral crests (fused trans processes), 4 post sacral foramina (for post rami of sacral Ns)
  - **Apex**: sacral hiatus

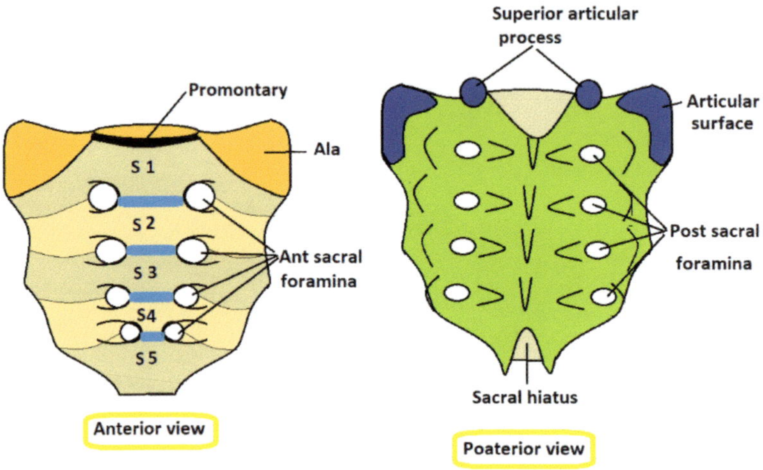

Figure 22: Anterior and posterior surfaces of the sternum

Thoracic cage

- Cone shaped cage
- Boundaries
  - **Ant**: sternum, costal cartilages
  - **Post**: vertebral column
  - **Lat**: ribs + intercostal spaces (muscles, Ns, Vessels)
  - **Inlet**: bounded by 1st rib + C1 vertebra + upper sternum
  - **Outlet**: Bounded by xiphoid process + costal margin + CC 11 & 12 + T 12 vertebra. Closed by the diaphragm.

Sternum (Fig. 23)

- **Manubrium**: articulates with the clavicle & 1st rib
  - Upper border: **suprasternal notch** (jugular notch) opposite the level of T2-T3 disc
  - **Sternal angle**: 2nd Costal Cartilage (used to identify the costal cartilages & ribs), present opposite T4-T5 disc
- **Body**: attachment of costal cartilages 2-7
- **Xiphoid process**: at level of T9, attachment of abdominal ms

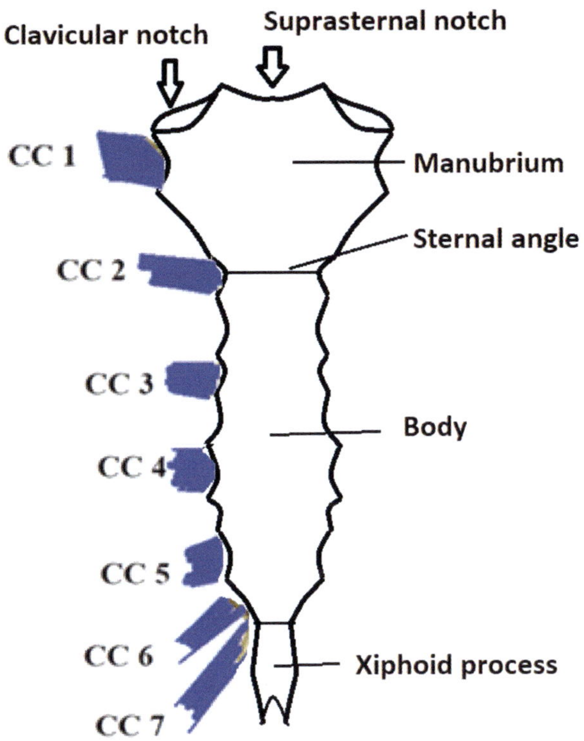

Figure 23: The sternum and the costal cartilages

<u>**Ribs**</u>

- 12 pairs, classified into (Fig. 24)
  - **True**: 1-7, attach to the sternum
  - **False**: 8-10, each attach to the one above
  - **Floating**: 11-12, are not attached
- **Costal margin**: formed by cost cartilages 7-10

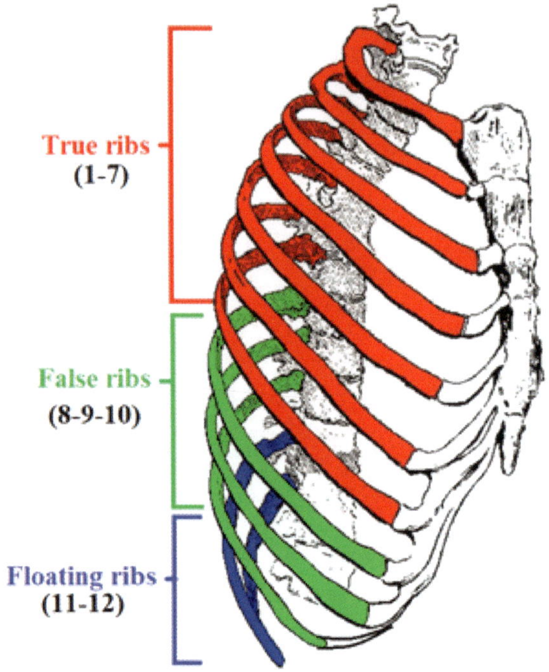

Figure 24: Classification of ribs

<u>Structure of rib</u> (Fig. 25)

- **Shaft**: have
  - costal groove (for intercostal N & Vessels)
  - inner & outer surfaces
  - rounded upper border
  - sharp lower border
- **Head**: articulates with body of same number vertebra & the body above
- **Neck**
- **Tubercle:** articulates with the transverse process of the same number vertebra
- **Ant end**: attaches to costal cartilage

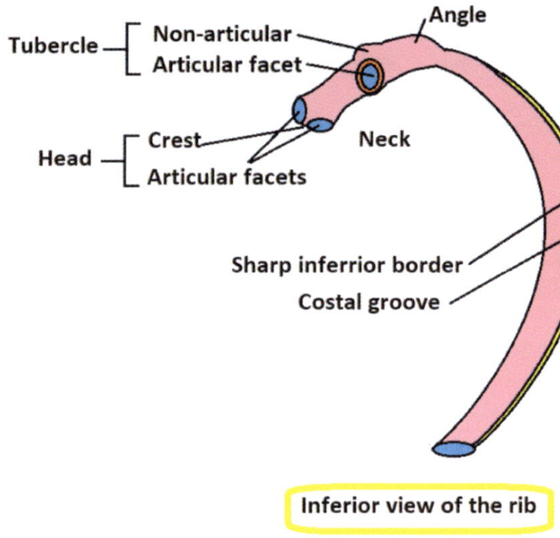

Figure 25: Structure of rib

Appendicular skeleton

Skeleton of Upper limb (Fig. 26)

- **Pectoral (shoulder) girdle:** Clavicle + scapula
- **Arm**: humerus
- **Forearm**: radius (lat) + ulna (med)
- **Hand**:
  - carpal bones (8)
  - metacarpals (5)
  - phalanges (5+5+4= 14)

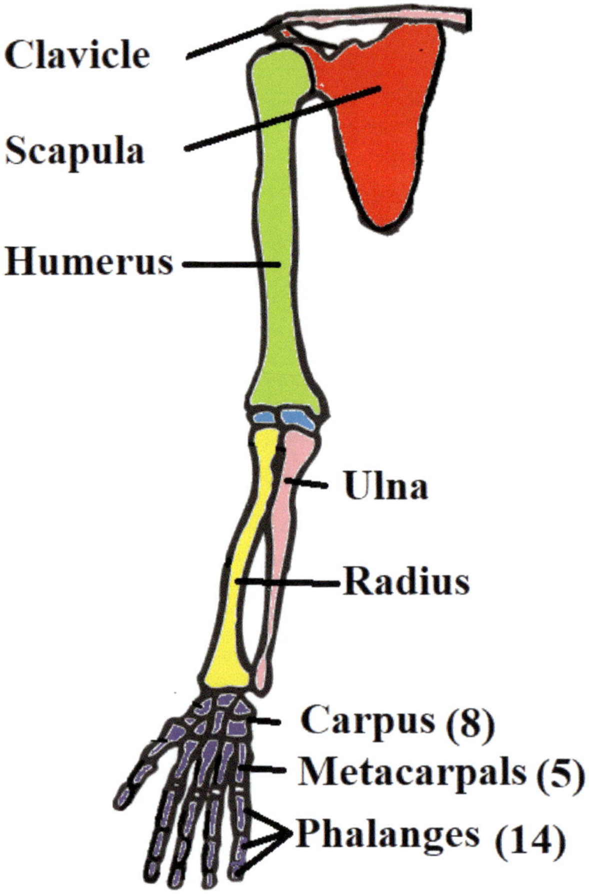

Figure 26: Skeleton of the upper limb

Pectoral (shoulder) girdle: Clavicle + scapula
Clavicle: shaft + 2 ends

- Sternal end: attached to manubrium
- Scapular end: attached to scapula
- Shaft: inf has trapezoid line & conoid tubercle

Scapula: triangular flat bone (Fig. 27)

- 3 borders: superior, lateral , medial
- 3 angles: lateral (glenoid cavity, forms shoulder joint), superior, inferior
- 2 surfaces
  - Ant surface: subscapular fossa
  - Post surface: spine (extends as the acromion process), supraspinous, infraspinous fossae

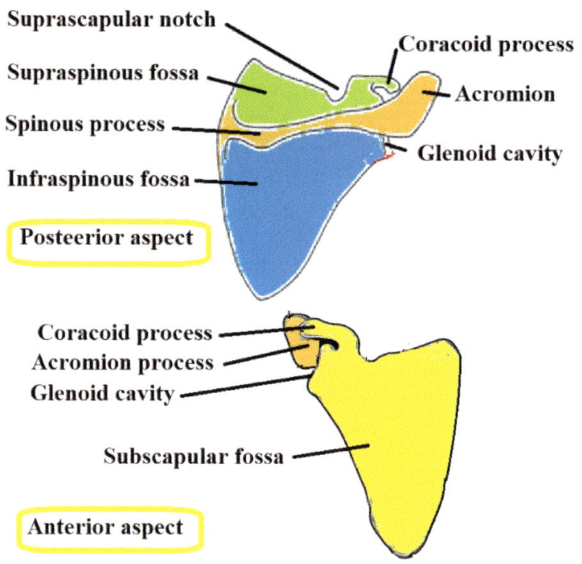

Figure 27: Scapula

<u>**Humerus**</u> (Fig. 28)
Upper end: Head, **neck** (anatomical & surgical), Greater & lesser tubercles, intertubercular groove

- Axillary N: passes around the **surgical neck**

Shaft: 3 borders, 3 surfaces, deltoid tuberosity

- Medial & lateral supracondylar ridges
- Radial N: passes in the **spiral groove**

Lower end: Trochlea, capitulum

- Ant: coronoid fossa (above trochlea), radial fossa (above capitulum)
- Post: Olecranon fossa (above trochlea)
- Lateral epicondyle
- **Medial** epicondyle (behind it passes the ulnar N)

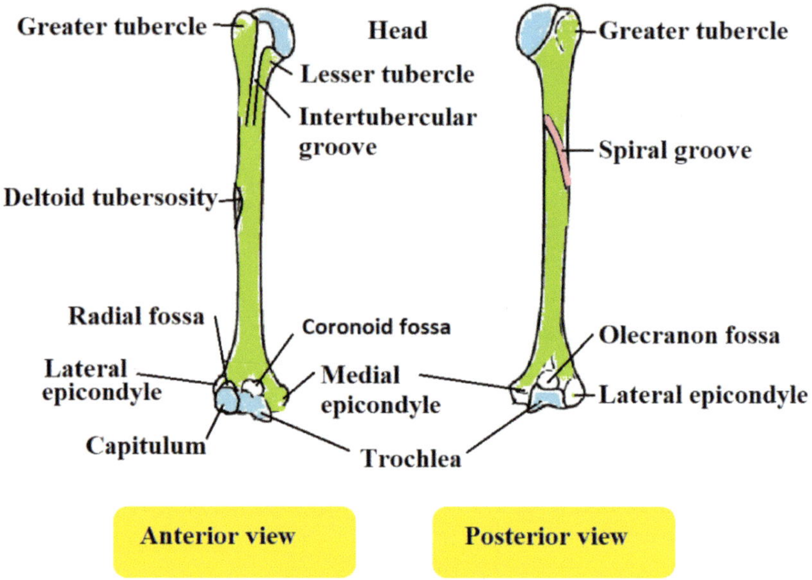

Figure 28: Humerus

Bones of the forearm

Radius (Fig. 29)

- Upper end: head, neck, radial tuberosity
- Shaft
- Lower end: styloid process (lat), ulnar notch (med)

Ulna (Fig. 24)

- Upper end:
  - 2 processes: olecranon (post), coronoid (ant)
  - 2 notches: trochlear (ant), radial (lat)
- Shaft:
- Lower end: Head, styloid process (med)

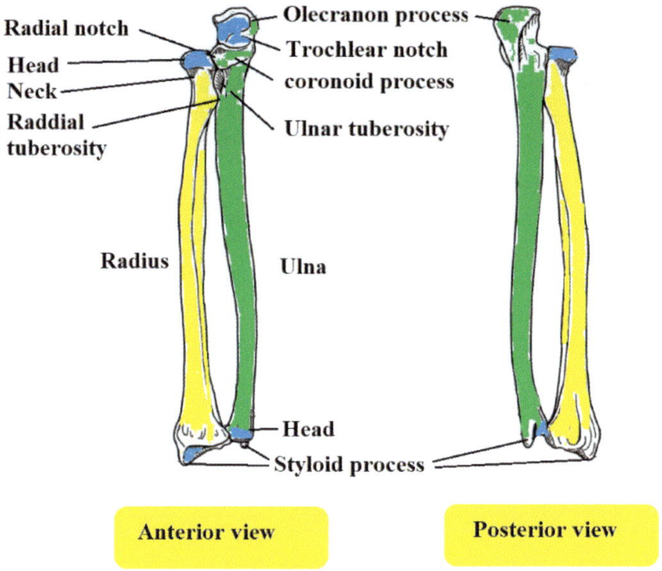

Figure 29: Radius and ulna

Hand

- **Carpus**: 2 rows (4+4) from lat to med
  - Proximal raw: **s**caphoid, **l**unate, **t**riquetrum, **p**isiform
  - Distal raw: **t**rapezium, **t**rapezoid, **c**apitate, **h**amate
  - Memory phrase: **S**ally **l**eft **t**he **p**arty **t**o **t**ake **C**indy **h**ome.
  - Concave ant forming the carpal tunnel
  - **Carpal tunnel syndrome**: compress median N (pain on the lat side of palm + weak thumb ms)
- **Metacarpus**: base, head, shaft
- **Phalanges**: 2 for thumb, 3 for each of the other fingers

Skeleton of lower limb (Fig. 30)

- **Pelvic girdle**: sacrum + hip bone
- **Thigh**: femur
- **Leg**: tibia + fibula
- **Foot**: tarsals + metatarsals + phalanges

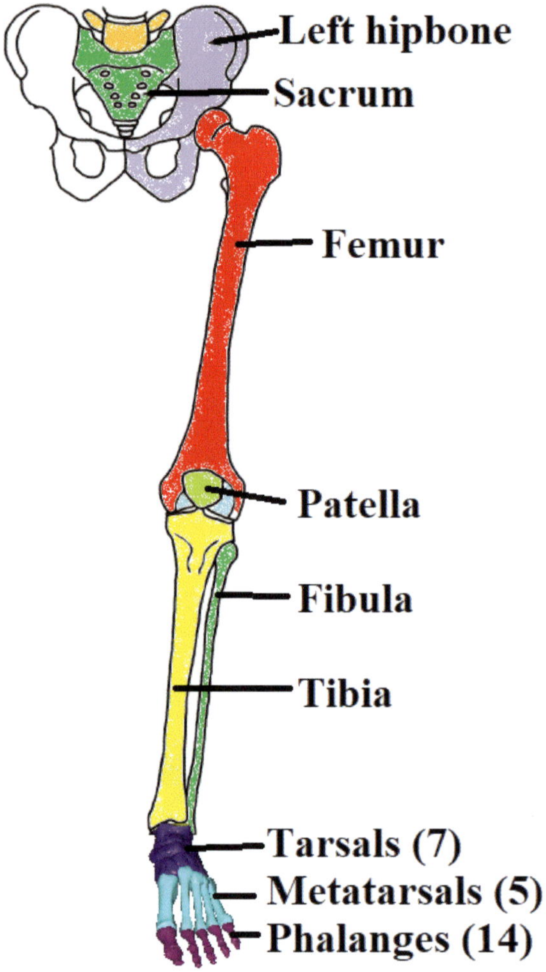

Figure 30: Skeleton of the lower limb

<u>Hip bone</u>

3 bones attached at the acetabulum (Fig. 31)

1) Ilium: body + ala

- Upper border: iliac crest, ASIS (ant), PSIS (post)
- Ant border: AIIS
- Post border: PIIS, greater sciatic notch
- Med surface: iliac fossa, auricular surface (articulate with sacrum)
- Lat surface: gluteal lines (ant, post, inf)

2) Ischium:

- Body: Ischial spine (med), lesser sciatic notch (post), Ischial tuberosity (post)
- Ramus:

3) Pubis:

- Body: upper border (pubic crest & tubercle), medial border (symphysis pubis)
- Superior ramus: obturator foramen
- Inferior ramus: pubic arch

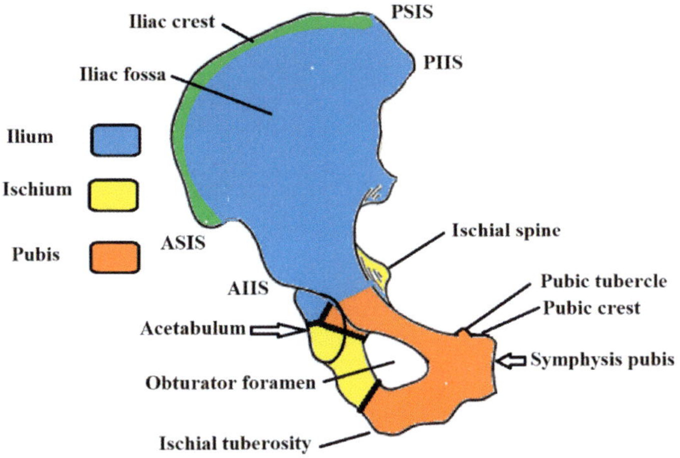

Figure 31: Hip bone

Gender differences of pelvis (Fig. 32)

Feature	**Female pelvis**	**Male pelvis**
Bones	Thin, smooth	Thick, prominent markings
Subpubic angle	Wide, 80-90 degrees	Acute, 50-60
Sacrum	Wide, short, less curved	Narrow, long, more curved
Greater sciatic notch	Wide, shallow	Narrow, deep
Pelvic inlet (brim)	Wide, oval	Narrow, heart-shaped
Pelvic outlet	Wide, ischial spines apart	Narrow, ischial spines point medially

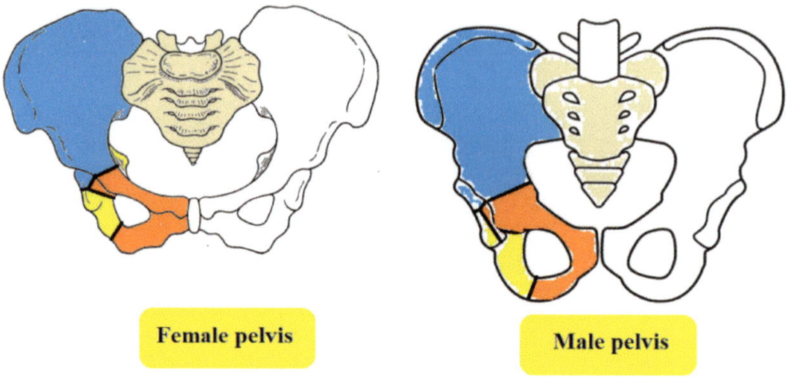

Figure 32: male and female pelvis

<u>**Femur**</u> (Fig. 33)

Upper end:

- Head: fovea capitis, attachment of lig of head of femur
- Neck: oblique, weak, could be fractured
- Greater trochanter
- Lesser trochanter
- Intertrochanteric line (ant)
- Intertrochanteric crest (post)

Shaft:

- gluteal tuberosity, linea aspera, med & lat supracondylar lines

Lower end:

- Lat & med condyles, intercondylar fossa & patellar surface
- Lat & med epicondyles, adductor tubercle

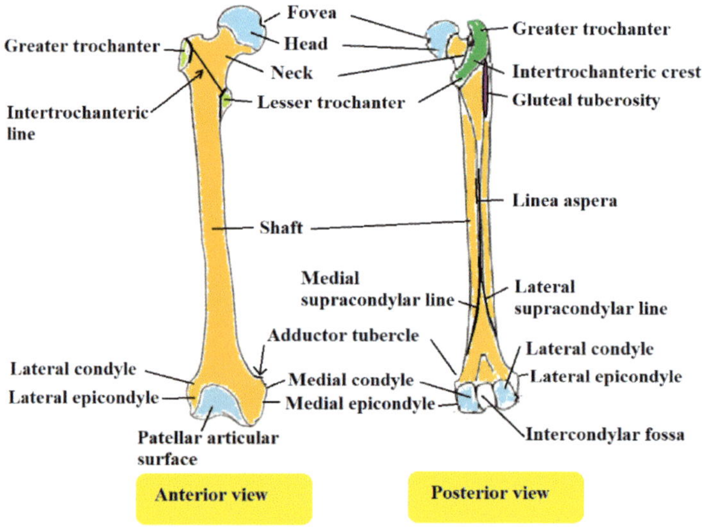

Figure 33: Femur

Tibia (Fig. 34)
Upper end:
- Med & lat condyles, intercondylar eminence
- Tibial tuberosity

Shaft: 3 borders (ant border is sharp), 3 surfaces (med surface is subcutaneous)
Lower end:
- med malleolus, fibular fossa

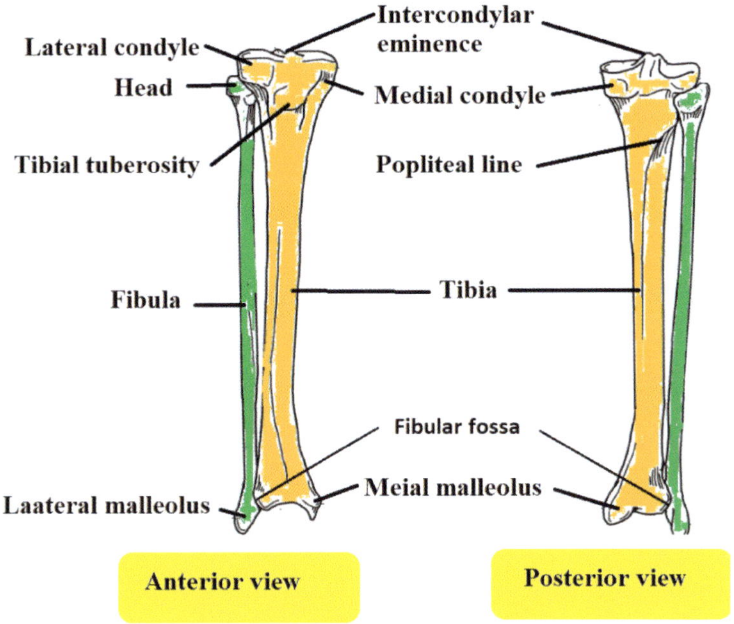

Figure 34: Tibia and fibula

Fibula (Fig. 34)
- Upper end: Head
- Shaft
- Lower end: lat malleolus

Foot
- **Tarsal bones**: Talus, calcaneus, navicular, cuboid, 3 cuneiform bones (med, intermediate, lat)
- **Metatarsal bones**: from 1 to 5
- **Phalanges**: 2 for the big toe, 3 for each of the other toes

Arches of the foot
- **Medial longitudinal arch**: is the highest arch, its failure is called **flat foot**

- Lateral longitudinal arch
- Transverse arch

Joints

Joint= articulation between 2 bones.

Types of Joints (Fig. 35)

I. Fibrous joints: bones connected by fibrous tissue, no movement

- Examples
  - Sutures of the skull
  - Interosseous membrane connecting radius & ulna, tibia & fibula
  - Articulation of tooth in its socket

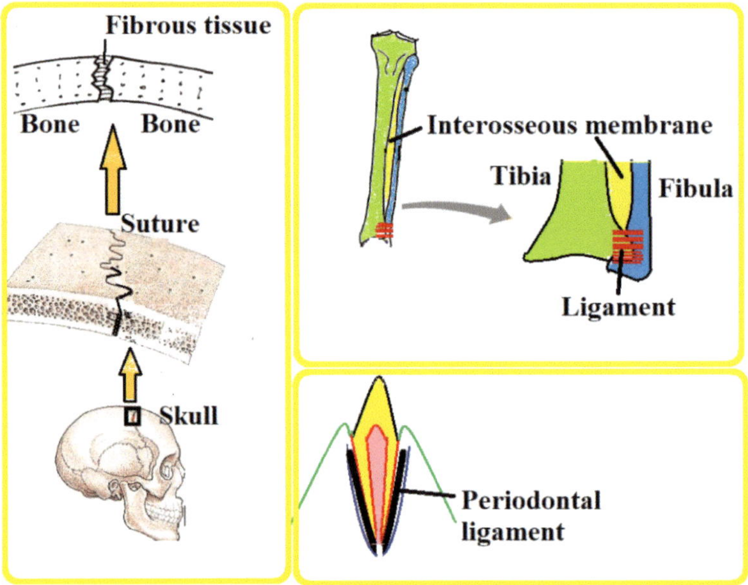

Figure 35: Fibrous joints

II. Cartilaginous joints: bones connected by cartilage, slightly movable

- Examples: (Fig. 36)
  - Symphysis pubis
  - Intervertebral discs
  - Epiphyseal plates

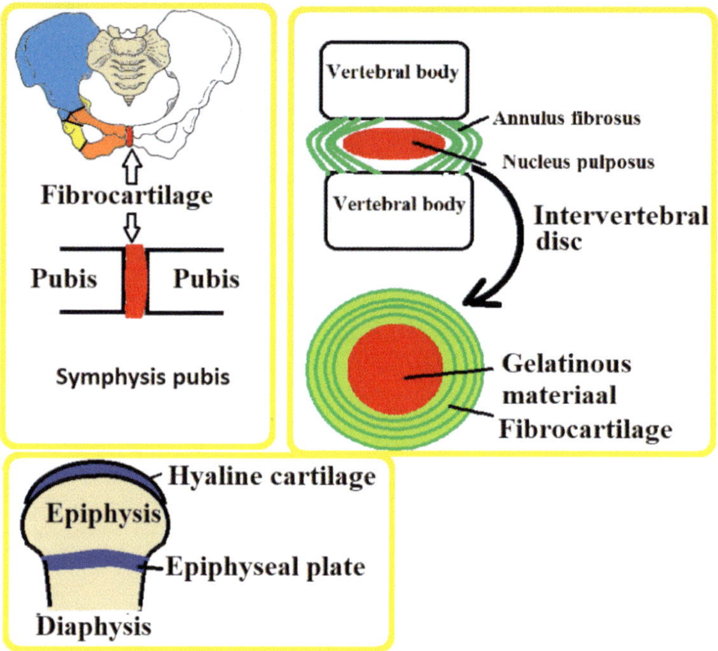

Figure 36: Cartilaginous joints

III. Synovial joints: Freely movable joint, bones are separated with joint cavity

Features of synovial joints:

- The 2 bones are covered with **articular cartilage**
- The 2 bones are connected with **capsule**
- The 2 bones are connected with **supporting ligaments**
- The 2 bones are separated with **joint cavity**
- The joint cavity is lined with **synovial membrane**, containing synovial fluid
- Have **nerve** supply and **vessels** supply

<u>Types of synovial joints</u>

Gliding type:

- Flat or slightly curved surfaces of bones
- Movement: Sliding or twisting
- *Examples*:
  - joints between the bones of the wrist
  - Joints between the bones of the ankle

<u>Movement in one axis</u>: pivot or hinge

- **Pivot joint:** (Fig. 37)
  - cylindrical part of one bone pivots within a ring

– Movement: rotation
– *Examples*:
  - Atlanto-axial joint.
  - proximal radio-ulnar joint

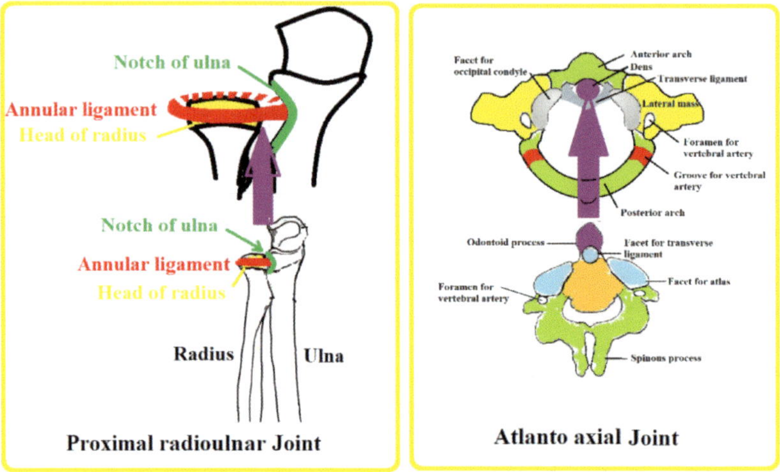

Figure 37: Synovial pivot joints

- **Hinge joint:** The convex surface of one bone articulates with the concave surface of another (Fig. 38).
  – Up and down movement in one plane is possible.
  – *Examples*: the elbow and knee joints.

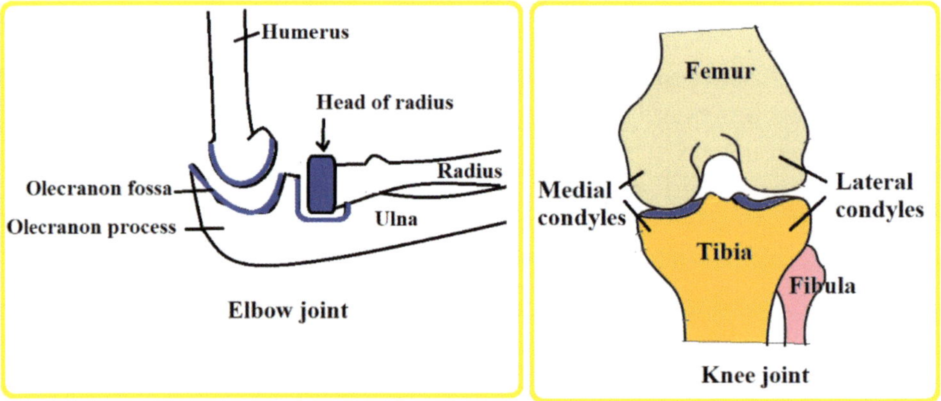

Figure 38: Hinge joints

<u>**Movement in 2 or more axes:**</u> condyloid, saddle, ball & socket

- **Condyloid joint:** oval-shaped condyle articulates with elliptical cavity
  – Movement in different planes is possible, except rotation
  – *Examples*: the metacarpo-phalangeal joints

- **Saddle joint:** Each bone is saddle-shaped
  - *Example*: the carpo-metacarpal joint of the thumb.

- **Ball-and-socket joint:** ball-shaped head fits into cup-shaped socket
  - Movements: in all planes + rotation
  - *Examples*: shoulder and hip joints (Fig. 39)

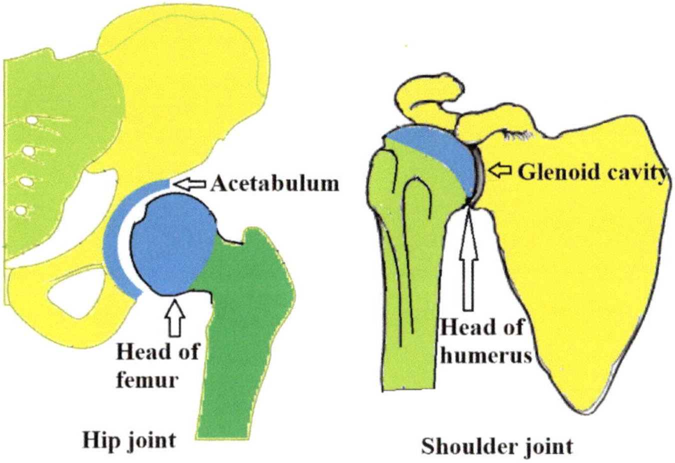

Figure 39: Ball & socket joints

<u>**Movements of Synovial Joints**</u>

- **Gliding**: articular surfaces are flat
- **Angular**
  - Movement in the sagittal plane: Flexion, extension (Fig. 40)

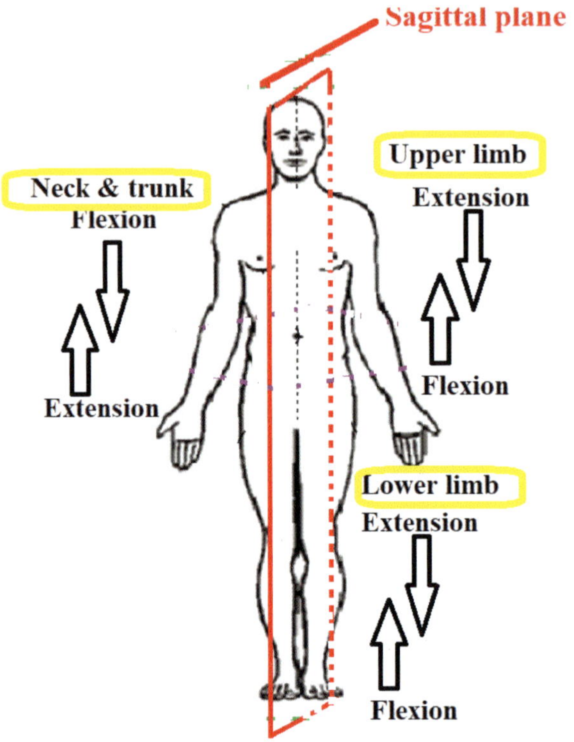

Figure 40: Flexion & extension

– Movement in the coronal plane: adduction, abduction (Fig. 41)

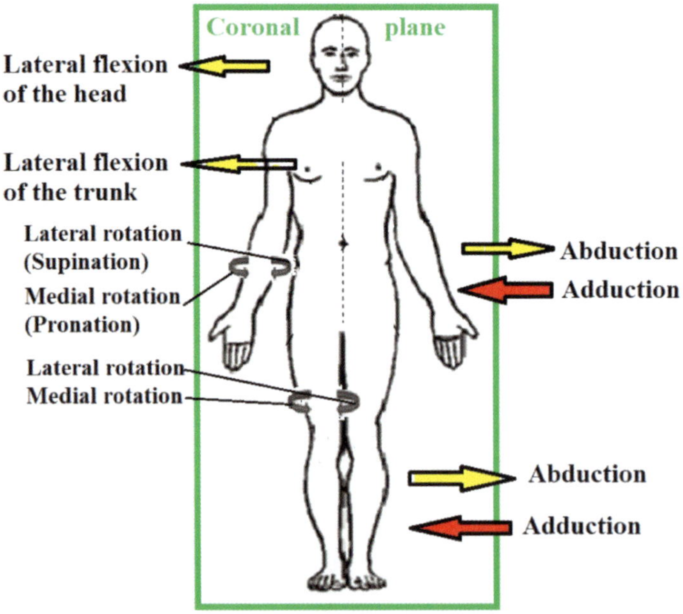

Figure 41: Adduction, abduction and rotation

- Circumduction= abduction, extension, adduction, flexion
- **Rotation**
  - Movement around the longitudinal axis
  - medial & lateral rotation (Fig. 41)
- **Special movements**
  - forearm: **supination** (palm faces ant), **pronation** (palm faces post)
  - foot:
    - ✓ **dorsiflexion** (toes face up), **plantarflexion** (toes face down)
    - ✓ **inversion** (sole faces inwards, **eversion**(sole faces outwards)
  - shoulder: **protraction** (forward movement), **retraction** (backward movement)
  - thumb: **opposition** (thumb opposes the other fingers)

Arthritis

- means joint damage
- can be caused by
  - overuse
  - chronic inflammation.

Osteoarthritis:

- Due to deterioration of the **articular cartilage** of a joint.
- caused by chronic overuse, older persons

Rheumatoid arthritis (RA)

- Inflammation of the **synovial membrane** → thicker cartilage.
- Caused by *autoimmune* reaction

Gout

- Due to increased **uric acid** in the blood
- Crystals of uric acid are deposited in the joints → inflammation.

Treatment:

- Analgesics
- Physical exercise
- chondrocyte implantation surgery
- Surgical replacement of the joint → followed by rehabilitation

Aging:

- Deterioration of cartilages & bones
- Cartilages calcify

Homeostasis of bones

- **Protect** the **internal organs** in thorax, abdomen, pelvis, skull and vertebral column.
- Protect **endocrine organs (**pituitary, pineal, and thymus).
- **Red bone marrow** → produces the RBCs (supply oxygen), WBCs (for immunity) and platelets (blood coagulation)
- store and release **calcium** (for muscles and nerves).
- help **digestion:** by chewing and breaking food

Chapter 4: Muscular system

A&P of skeletal muscles

Types of muscles

- **Three types** of muscle tissue: skeletal, cardiac, smooth

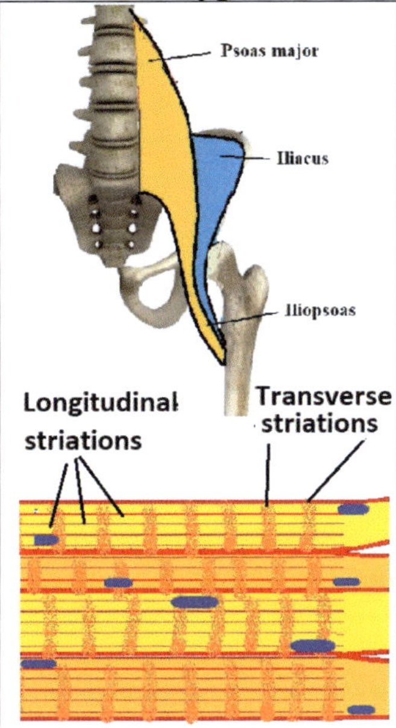

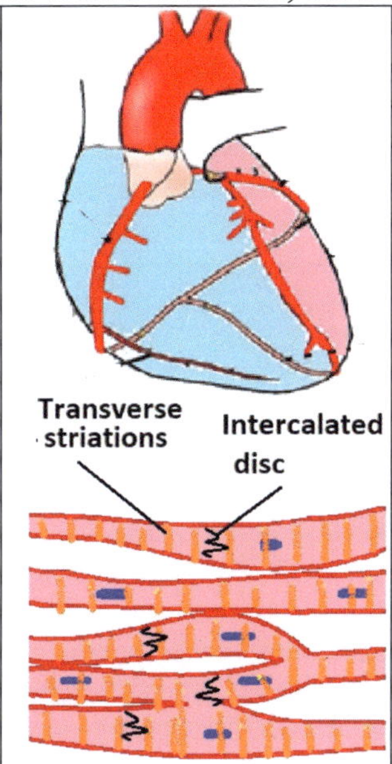

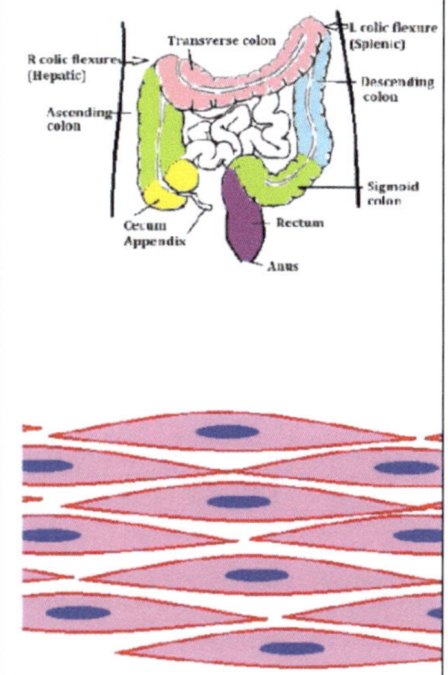

Skeletal muscle	**Cardiac muscle**	**Smooth muscle**
striated, cylindrical, Multinucleated fibers	striated, cylindrical, branched fibers, with one or two nuclei	spindle-shaped fibers, with single nucleus
Location: attached to skeleton or skin	**Location**: heart walls	**Location**: walls of hollow organs (e.g., stomach, intestines, urinary bladder, uterus, blood vessels)
NS: somatic	**NS:** autonomic	**NS:** autonomic
Control: voluntary	**Control**: involuntary	**Control**: involuntary

Connective tissue of skeletal muscles (Fig. 1)

- **Endomysium:** surrounds each fiber
- **Perimysium:** surrounds the muscle bundles (*fascicles)*
- **Epimysium:** surrounds the whole muscle
  - The epimysium blends with the ***deep fascia***.

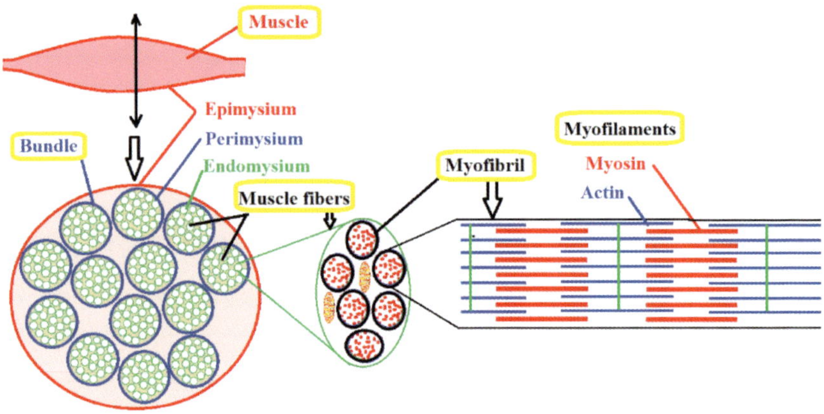

Figure 1: Structure of the muscle and its connective tissue

Deep fascia

- Separates muscles from each other and from the **superficial fascia** (hypodermis).
- Surrounds a group of muscles = **muscle compartment**.
- **Compartment syndrome:** → is increased tension inside the compartment → obstructing the blood supply to the muscles.

Functions of skeletal muscles

- **Move** bones and body parts (like eye, face & thorax)
- **protect** internal organs, bones, joints
- **support** body by contracting against gravity
- assists **fluid movement** in cardiovascular and lymphatic vessels
- maintain constant body **temperature**

Structure of muscle fiber

- Have alternating **light and dark bands** → give *striated* (striped) appearance.
- Bands are due to alternating **actin** and **myosin** filaments.
- plasma membrane is called ***sarcolemma***
- cytoplasm is called ***sarcoplasm***
- smooth endoplasmic reticulum is called ***sarcoplasmic reticulum***

Level of organization in skeletal muscle:

- **Muscle**, consists of
- **Muscle fiber**: extends along the entire length of the muscle
- **Myofibril**: extends along the entire length of the muscle
- Consists of **2 protein contractile elements**: (Fig. 2)
  - **thick filaments = myosin**

- **thin filaments = actin**

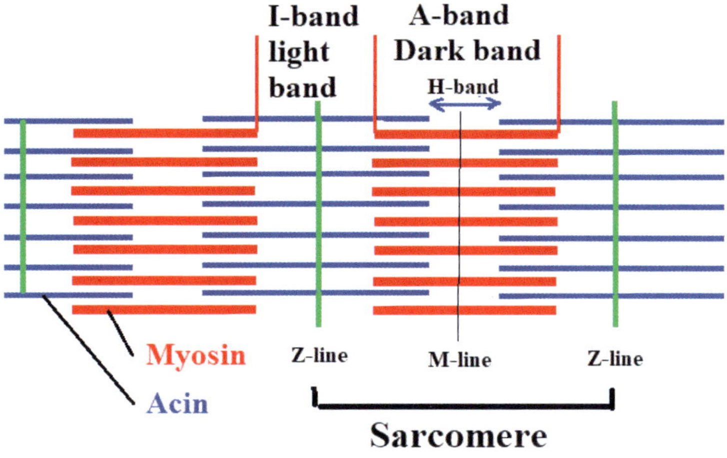

Figure 2: Sarcomere

<u>**Electron Microscopic structure**</u> (Fig. 2)
Shows alternating **dark bands** (**A** bands) and **light bands** (**I** bands)

- **A** band
  - Mainly **thick filaments (myosin)**
  - **Thin filaments** overlaps it, except in the H zone
  - **H zone** at its middle
  - **M line** at the middle of the H zone
- **I** band
  - **Thin filaments (actin)** only
  - **Z line** in its middle
- **Sarcomere**: (Fig. 2)
  - the part of the myofibril between two Z lines
  - it is the functional unit of skeletal muscle.
  - Cross bridges extend from the thick filaments
- **Titin:** (Fig. 3)
  - highly elastic protein
  - extend from the M line to the Z lines
  - is the largest protein in the body
  - contributes to the muscle's elasticity

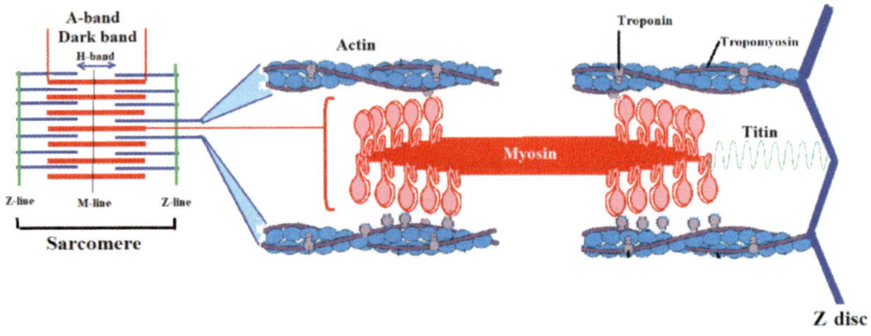

Figure 3: The contractile elements of the skeletal muscle

<u>**Myosin thick filament**</u> (Figs. 3 & 4)

- Consists of **two** identical subunits, each shaped like a **golf club** (with head + tail).
- **The heads** form the **cross bridges**, each with two sites:
  - actin binding site
  - Myosin ATPase site.
- **The tail** ends are intertwined around each other, and directed toward the center of the filament

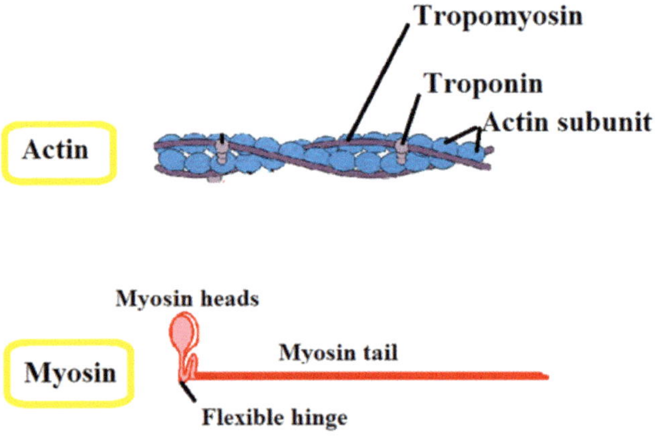

Figure 4: Structure of actin & myosin

<u>**Thin filament**</u>

Consists of **3 proteins**: (Fig. 4)

1) Actin

- **Spherical protein molecules** arranged into **two strands,** twisted to form a spiral

- Each molecule has a special binding site for a **myosin cross bridge**

2) Tropomyosin molecules

- **Threadlike proteins** that lie alongside the grooves of the actin spiral.
- Covers the sites of the cross bridges.

3) Troponin: have **three binding sites:**

- one binds to **tropomyosin**
- one binds to **actin**
- one can bind to **calcium (Ca^{2+})**

<u>The mechanism of muscle contraction</u>

(a) In relaxed muscle, tropomyosin covers myosin binding sites on actin.
(b) When **Ca^{2+}** is released → it binds to **troponin** → the shape of troponin changes → **tropomyosin** slips away → **exposing myosin binding sites** → myosin binds to actin at the **cross bridges** → **ATP** triggers the cross bridges to **bend** (**Sliding Filament Mechanism**) → Cross-bridges form, bend, then break and reform → a **power stroke** causes actin to move at the sarcomere → **shortens** the myofibril.

<u>Sliding Filament Mechanism</u> (Fig. 5)

- The **thin filaments** on each side of a sarcomere **slide inward** over the stationary thick filaments toward its center
- The **Z lines are pulled** closer together → shortens the following:
  - **Sarcomere** → shortens the entire fiber
  - **H zone** shortens
  - **I band** shortens
- The width of the A band remains unchanged.
- The thick or thin filaments do not decrease in length.

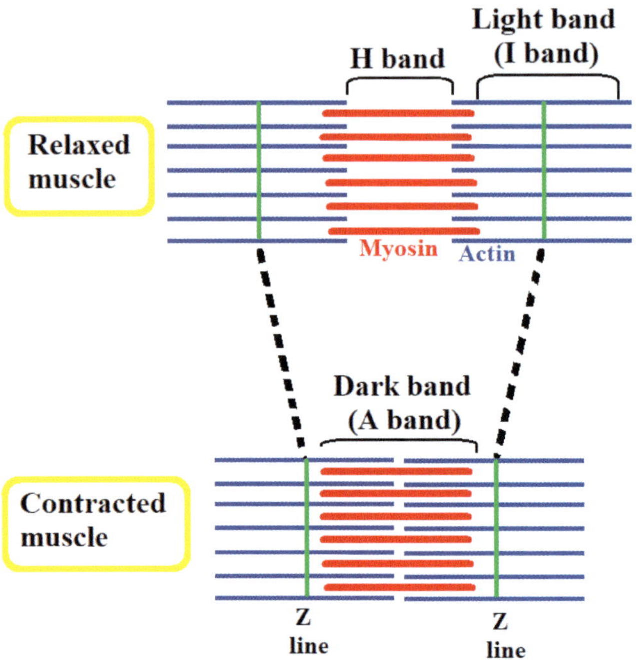

Figure 5: Contracted & relaxed muscle

Power stroke (Fig. 3)

- A single **cross-bridge interaction cycle**, include the following:
  - **Binding:** Myosin cross bridge binds to actin molecule.
  - **Power stroke:** Cross bridge **bends**, pulling thin myofilament inward.
  - **Detachment:** Cross bridge detaches and returns to its original conformation.
  - **Binding** of cross bridge to a **more distal actin molecule** → cycle is repeated.

T-tubules (transverse tubule) (Fig. 6)

- Present at the junction of A band and I band
- the surface membrane dips into the muscle fiber to form **T tubule**

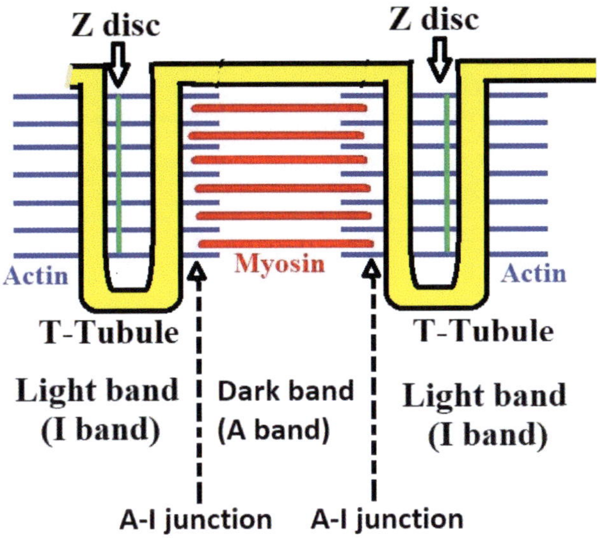

Figure 6: T-tubule

Excitation contraction Coupling

1) Action potential arrives → spreads down the **T tubule** →
2) triggers **release of Ca^{++}** from the sarcoplasmic reticulum.
3) Ca^{++} binds to **troponin** →
4) Tropomyosin moves away, uncovering the **binding site** →
5) Myosin **cross bridges** attach to the binding sites →
6) ATP triggers the cross bridges to **bend** →
7) Fresh ATP binds to myosin cross bridge → Cross bridge **detach** from actin → ATP is hydrolyzed (cycle is repeated).

Role of Ca^{++} in the cross bridges

- Ca^{2+} is the link between excitation (**action potential**) and contraction (**cross bridge bending).**

(a) Relaxed muscle

- No cross-bridge binding
- Muscle fiber is relaxed

(b) Excited muscle

- → **Ca^{2+} is released** → **Ca^{2+} binds with troponin** → pulling troponin–tropomyosin complex aside to expose cross-bridge binding site → **Cross-bridge binding occurs** → **triggers power stroke** that pulls thin filament inward during contraction

Types of contraction

- **Isotonic contraction** = constant tension, while the muscle length changes
- **Isometric contraction** = constant length, while tension develops at constant muscle length

Rigor Mortis: no fresh ATP available (after death), actin and myosin remain bound in rigor complex, due to:
- Cross bridges **cannot detach** from actin
- also **Ca^{++} increase** in cytosol

Cardiac & smooth muscles

Cardiac muscle
- Similar to skeletal muscle, but has **no T-tubules**
- **Ca^{++}** comes from outside the cell as well as inside.
- After the action potential signal → **Ca^{++}** diffuses into the sarcoplasm → triggers the release of more **Ca^{++}** from the sarcoplasmic reticulum.
- **Ca^{++}** binds to **troponin** → **cross-bridges** form between activated myosin and actin.

Smooth muscle
- does **not have Z lines**
- but have **dense bodies** containing the same protein of Z lines
- **actin filaments** are attached to the dense bodies.
- When a smooth muscle cell contracts → its fibers shorten in all directions → become more oval in shape.
- During excitation, the increased smooth muscle **Ca^{++}** → binds with **calmodulin** (which is similar to troponin).
- The Ca^{++} / calmodulin complex → initiates **phosphorylation** of the **myosin light chain** → binds with **actin** → **cross-bridge cycling** begins.
- Contraction is slow, but last long without fatigue.

Energy for Muscle Contraction

3 steps in contraction–relaxation process **require ATP**:
1. **power stroke** of the cross bridge.
2. bridge **detach** from actin
3. Active transport of **Ca^{++} back**

<u>3 pathways</u> to supply ATP (Fig. 7)

1) **ADP + Creatine phosphate → ATP +Creatine**

2) **<u>Oxidative phosphorylation</u>** (cellular respiration).

   – Occur in the **mitochondria**.
   – Depends on delivery of **adequate O_2** & nutrients.
   – Is **aerobic** ("needs O_2") or **endurance- type exercise.**
      • **Glucose + O_2 + ADP → ATP + CO_2 + water**

3) **<u>Fermentation</u>**

- Occurs without **O_2 (anaerobic)**
- Occurs in the **sarcoplasm**
- **Glucose + ADP → ATP + Lactate** (lactic acid)
- → lactate accumulation → gives the sense of fatigue & pain
- → **Cramping** = the inability of a muscle to completely relax
   – is due to lack of ATP

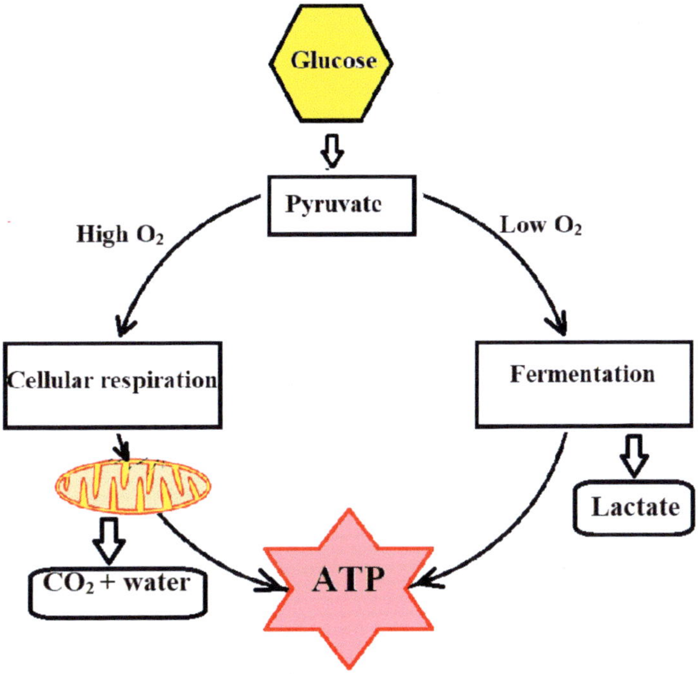

Figure 7: ATP supply to the skeletal muscles

- **oxidative phosphorylation** → yields **32 ATP**
- **Anaerobic glycolysis** → yields **2 ATP**
   – Produces **lactate** → leads to **fatigue, pain and stiff ness** → produces metabolic acidosis (fall in muscle pH)
   – can be sustained for a short duration
- **During exercise**
   – **Creatine phosphate** stores are reduced

- **lactate** accumulate
- **Glycogen** re depleted
- body **temperature** rises
- **Oxygen debt** is created when a muscle uses **fermentation** to supply energy.

- **During recovery** from exercise → excess oxygen consumption, is due to various factors.
  - Repayment of **oxygen debt** (ATP)
    - replenishing creatine phosphate supplies
    - Disposing lactic acid
  - elevated secretion of **epinephrine**

Muscle response

- **threshold stimulus** = a **stimulus** strong enough to lead to muscle contraction
- **muscle twitch** = single contraction followed by relaxation
  - It is recorded by **myogram**

<u>A muscle twitch has 3 stages</u>: (Fig. 8)

1) The **latent period** is the interval between the threshold stimulus and the onset of the muscle contraction.
   - **Acetylcholine** diffuses across the neuromuscular junction → binds to receptors on the muscle → **action potential** spreads → **Ca^{++}** is released from the sarcoplasmic reticulum.

2) The **contraction period:**
   - cross-bridges are formed
   - Thick and thin myofilaments slide over each other.
   - The muscle shortens
   - Force is generated

3) The **relaxation period**:
   - Cross-bridges break
   - **Ca^{++}** is returned to the sarcoplasmic reticulum.
   - The muscle returns to its previous length

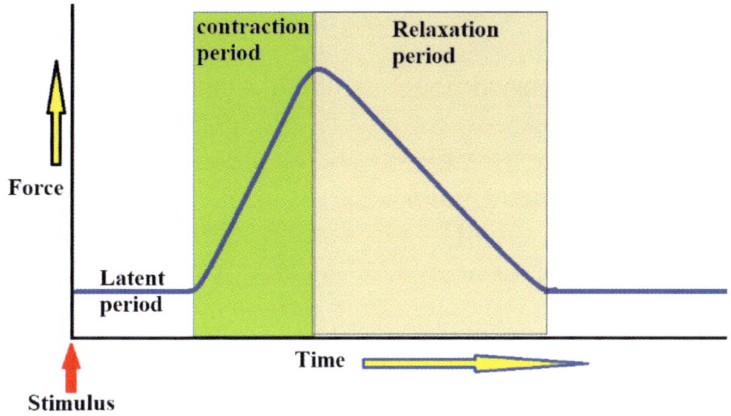

Figure 8: Stages of the muscle twitch

<u>Summation</u> (Fig. 9)

- Series of stimuli → produces series of muscle twitches.
- the muscle is stimulated rapidly → giving greater contraction force
  - there is no enough time between stimuli to return all the **Ca**$^{++}$ to the sarcoplasmic reticulum → leading to more cross-bridges after each stimulus.
  - It generates heat

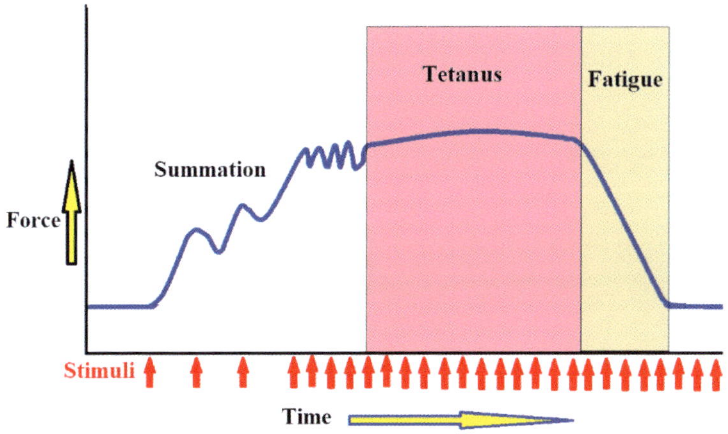

Figure 9: Summation, tetanus and fatigue of skeletal muscle

<u>Tetanus</u> (tetanic contraction) (Fig. 9)

- Occurs when the muscle is stimulated very rapidly → the muscle has no time to relax → the muscle force becomes more and more constant.
- → It will continue until the muscle **fatigues.**
- It differs from the disease **tetanus** which is caused by bacteria

Fatigue: (Fig. 9)

- The muscle relaxes although stimulation continues.
- **Causes of fatigue**:
  - Depletion of **ATP**
  - production of **lactic acid**
  - lowering the **pH** → leading to acidic sarcoplasm
  - Depletion of **acetylcholine** from the motor nerves
- Intact muscles in the body rarely fatigue.

Motor units in skeletal muscles

- **motor unit** = one motor neuron + all the muscle fibers innervated by it (Fig. 10)
- It functions according to the **all-or-none law**
- **One motor neuron** innervates a number of muscle fibers, but **each muscle fiber** is supplied by only one motor neuron.
- For muscles that produce **precise, delicate movements,** (eye and hands muscles), a single motor unit supply few fibers (23 muscle fibers or lower)
- For muscles that produce **powerful, coarse movements**, (as the legs) a single motor unit supply large number of muscle fibers (1000 to 2000)
- **muscle tone**: some muscle fibers are always contracting.
  - is important in maintaining **posture**.

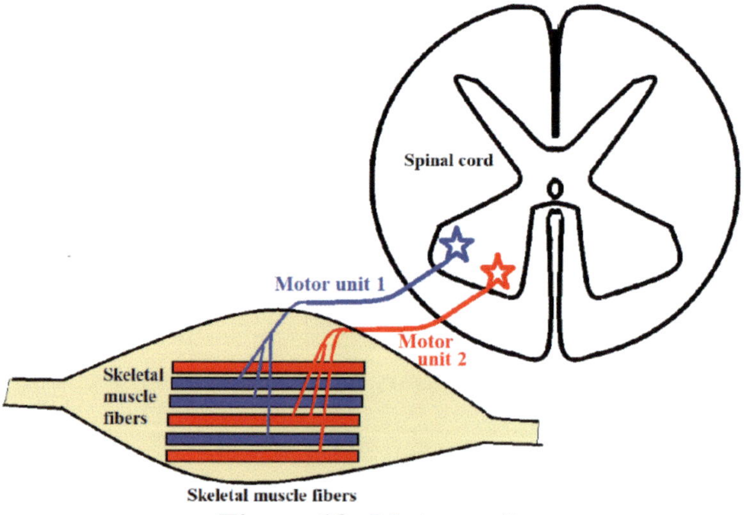

Figure 10: Motor units

Size of Muscles

- **Atrophy** (= decrease in the size of the muscle fiber)

  - occurs in muscles that are not used or used for very weak contractions
  - Examples: limb in cast or nerve damage
- **Hypertrophy** (= increase in size of the muscle fiber)
  - Occurs only if the muscle contracts to at least 75% of its maximum tension over a prolonged period.

Types of muscle fibers

Most muscles contain mixture of 2 types of fibers

1) Slow-oxidative fibers (Type I)

- **Aerobic** muscle fibers
- **slow** contractions for **long periods** without fatigue
- Example: the muscles of the **back and legs**
- more likely to succeed in **endurance activities** (as **marathon races)**
- Are rich in mitochondria
- Richly supplied with capillaries
- have **high myoglobin** content (store small amounts of O_2)
  - gives the muscle red color (Called **red fibers)**
- Have a greater capacity to form ATP
- There is no lactate accumulation
- More resistant to fatigue.

2) Fast-glycolytic fibers (Type II)

- **Anaerobic** muscle fibers
- **rapid** movements for **short period**
- Example: the **arm** muscles
- Respond to **resistance training** (as **power and sprint events)**
- Have **higher myosin ATPase** (ATP-splitting) activity
  - Contains a lot of stored **glycogen**
  - contains little myoglobin
  - are pale in color, so they are called **white fibers**
- Two factors determine the speed of muscle
  - **Load** (load–velocity relationship)
  - **ATPase activity** (fast or slow **twitch**)

<u>Twitch of Muscle Fibers</u>

- **Slow-twitch** muscle fibers
  - provide myofibrils with ATP **aerobically** (using O2)
  - **type I** fibers: Slow-twitch- **Aerobic**
  - **type IIa** fibers: are intermediate-twitch- **Aerobic**

- **Fast- twitch** muscle fibers
    - are **anaerobic** (using fermentation or creatine phosphate).
    - **type IIb** fibers: are fast-twitch- **Anaerobic**

Adaptation of muscle fibers

2 types of adaptation changes occur:

1) Improvement of the **oxidative capacity**
    - Achieved by regular **aerobic** **endurance exercise** (as long-distance **jogging** or **swimming)**
    - Mechanism: increase in the number of **mitochondria** and **capillaries** → the muscle uses O_2 more efficiently
2) **Hypertrophy (**Increase in **diameter)** of muscle fibers
    - Achieved by regular **anaerobic**, short-duration, high intensity **resistance training** (as **weight-lifting) → hypertrophy** of the **fast-glycolytic fibers**
    - **testosterone** promotes the synthesis of actin and myosin filaments (is a dangerous practice)

Muscular disorders

Rigor mortis = stiffness of death

- **Forensic pathologists** use it to determine the time of death.
    - It starts 3h after death
    - become full 8 hs
    - resolves 24–36 hours after death
- It occurs because of **depletion** of **ATP**.
- ATP energy is needed to
    - Break the bond between an actin binding site and the myosin cross-bridge.
    - Return Ca^{++} ions from the sarcoplasm to the sarcoplasmic reticulum
- Without ATP, the muscle remains fixed in contraction that preceded death of the person.

Abnormal contractions:

- **Spasms:** sudden, involuntary muscular **contractions** of smooth or skeletal muscle, and are often painful.
- **Convulsions:** Multiple **spasms** of skeletal muscles
- **Cramp:** are strong, **painful spasms**, especially of the leg and foot, usually due to strenuous athletic activity.

- **Tics:** are **spasms** that can be controlled voluntarily with great effort (as periodic eye blinking or grimacing)
- **Strain:** caused by stretching or tearing of a muscle
- **Sprain:** twisting of a **joint**, leading to swelling and injury of muscles, ligaments and tendons
- **Tendinitis:** is inflammation of a **tendon** due to repeated strong activity.

<u>**Neuromuscular Diseases**</u>

- **Tetanus**: secretes **toxin** that inhibit muscle contractions.
- **Fibromyalgia** is a chronic condition of **muscle ache**, tenderness, and stiffness.
- **Muscular dystrophy** is a group of disorders that cause progressive degeneration and **weakening** of muscles.
- **Duchenne muscular dystrophy**
  - Is the most common type of muscle dystrophy
  - → it affects only boys
  - is carried by the mother.
- **Myasthenia gravis**
  - is an **autoimmune disease**
  - → produces antibodies → destroy **acetylcholine receptors** on the sarcolemma
  - Causes muscle weakness in the head, neck, limbs.
- **Multiple sclerosis (MS)**
  - is an **autoimmune disease**
  - attacks myelin sheath
  - muscle weakness, paralysis, double vision, and dizziness.
- **Amyotrophic lateral sclerosis (ALS) = Lou Gehrig's disease**:
  - → gradual death of motor neurons
  - → lose the ability to walk, talk, chew, swallow, etc.
  - Intellect and sensation are not affected.

<u>**Motor abnormalities**</u>

- **Spastic paralysis**
  - Due to loss of inhibitory fibers
  - → **increased muscle tone** and **augmented limb reflexes**
- **Flaccid paralysis**
  - due to loss of descending excitatory tracts
  - **Muscles are relaxed**
  - Loss of **voluntary muscle contraction**
  - **Spinal reflex** activity is still present.
  - **Hemiplegia**:

- flaccid paralysis of the opposite half of the body
    - Due to damage of the primary motor cortex on one side of the brain (as in stroke)
  - **Paraplegia**:
    - paralysis of the legs
    - Due to lower-spinal-cord injury.
  - **Quadriplegia**
    - paralysis of the 4 limbs
    - Due to disruption of all descending pathways
    - as in the damaged in upper-spinal-cord
  - Destruction of **lower motor neurons** (cell bodies or efferent motor fibers)
    - Leads to flaccid paralysis and lack of reflexes
- Damage to the **cerebellum or basal nuclei**
  - Gives uncoordinated, clumsy activity and inappropriate patterns of movement.
  - There is no paralysis
- Damage to **higher cortical regions**
  - Gives inability to establish conscious motor commands

Basic anatomical principles of skeletal muscles

Muscle attachment

- **origin** is the stationary end
- **insertion** is the mobile end

Muscle movements

- **prime mover = agonist:** the main muscle for a movement
- **synergist**: the assisting muscle
- **Antagonist**: the opposite muscle
- ***Example***: in flexing the forearm at the elbow:
  - prime mover is the **brachialis**
  - synergist is the **biceps brachii**
  - Antagonist is the **triceps brachii** → it extends the forearm

Muscle action

- **flexion** is a movement that decreases the angle at a joint
- **extension** is a movement that increases the angle at a joint.
- **abduction** is a movement away from the midline
- **adduction** is a movement toward the midline.
- **rotation** is the movement of a part around its own axis.

Naming Muscles

Uses the following terms

- 1. **Size**. For example:
  - *gluteus* ***maximus*** is the largest muscle in the buttocks.
  - *gluteus minimus* is the smallest of the gluteal muscles.
  - *vastus* (huge)
  - *longus* (long)
  - *brevis* (short)
- 2. **Shape**. For example
  - *deltoid* is shaped like delta, or triangle
  - *trapezius* is shaped like a trapezoid
  - *latissimus* (wide)
  - *teres* (rounded).
- 3. **Direction of fibers**. For example
  - *rectus abdominis* (*rectus* means straight).
  - *orbicularis oculi* is around the eye.
  - *transverse* (across) and *oblique* (diagonal).
- 4. **Location**. For example
  - *frontalis* overlies the frontal bone.
  - *external oblique* is located outside the internal oblique.
  - *pectoralis* (chest)
  - *gluteus* (buttock)
  - *brachii* (arm)
  - *sub* (beneath)
- 5. **Attachment**. For example
  - *sternocleidomastoid* is attached to the sternum, clavicle, and mastoid process.
  - *Brachioradialis* is attached to the brachium (arm) and the radius.
- 6. **Number of attachments**. For example
  - *biceps brachii* has two origins (*bi* = 2)
  - *quadriceps femoris* has four origins (*quad* = 4)
- 7. **Action**. For example
  - *extensor digitorum* extends the fingers or digits.
  - *adductor magnus* adducts the thigh.
  - *flexor* (to flex)
  - *masseter* (to chew)
  - *levator* (to elevate)

Skeletal Muscle Groups

- The muscles are **grouped** according to their location and action.
- **Location**: note the following:

- **arm** refers to the humeral area
- **forearm***: refers to* radius/ulna area
- **Thigh***: refers to* the femur area
- **leg***: refers to* the tibia/fibular area

• **Action**: movement could be known from the origin and insertion

Abbreviations

- *O: origin*
- *I: insertion*
- *NS: nerve supply*
- *N: nerve*
- *CN: cranial nerve*
- *CC: costal cartilages*

Muscles of head & neck

Muscles of facial expression

1) Are located on the scalp and face.
2) They show the expressions of surprise, angry, fear, happy, etc.
3) **O**: from bone or skin
4) **I**: into skin.
5) **Action**: moves skin → gives facial expressions
6) **Nerve supply**: facial N (CN 7)

They include (Fig. 11)

1) **Occipito-frontalis**:
   - **2 frontal bellies**:
     - ➢ lie over the frontal bone
     - ➢ raise the eyebrows and wrinkle the brow
     - ➢ Frequent use → gives furrowing of the forehead
   - **2 occipital bellies**:
     - ➢ lie over the occipital bone
   - **epicranial aponeurosis**: connects the 4 bellies
2) **Orbicularis oculi** encircles the eye.
   - It closes the eye → blinking.
3) **Orbicularis oris** encircles the mouth
   - Puckers the lips → as in forming a kiss.

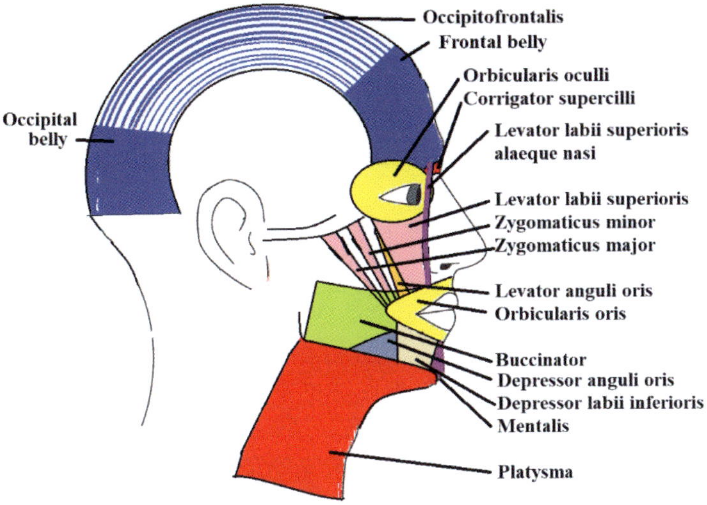

Figure 11: Muscles of facial expression

4) **Buccinator**: It is called the "**trumpeter's muscle**."
   - Is located in the cheek.
   - **Action**:
     - ➢ It compresses the cheek, as in whistling or blowing out air.
     - ➢ Holds food in contact with the teeth during chewing.
     - ➢ Babies use this muscle for suckling.
5) **Zygomaticus minor & major** extends from each zygomatic arch (cheekbone) to the corners of the mouth.
   - They raise the corners of the mouth in smiling.
6) **Levator anguli oris** and **levator labii superioris** lift the upper edge and corners of the lip, as in smiling.
7) **Depressor anguli oris** and **depressor labii inferioris** pull the corners of the lip down, as in frowning.
8) **Platysma:** in the neck

<u>Muscles of mastication</u>

1) **Masseter**: (Fig. 12)
   - O: zygomatic arch
   - I: angle of mandible
   - Action: elevates the mandible
2) **Temporalis**: (Fig. 12)
   - O: temporal fossa
   - I: coronoid process of mandible
   - Action: elevates the mandible

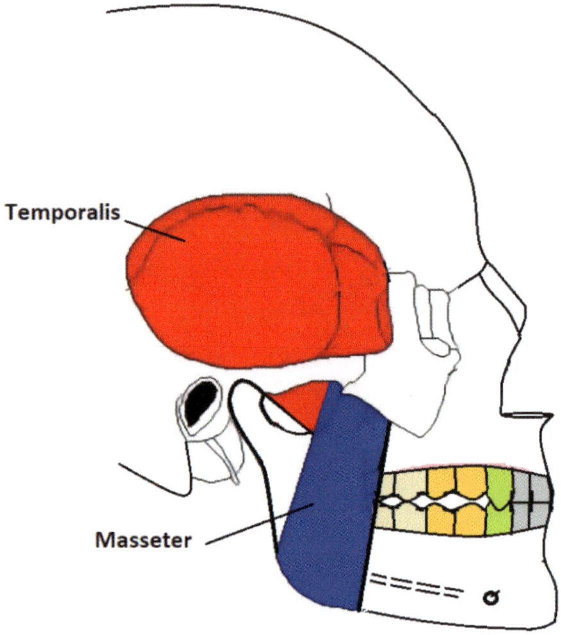

Figure 12: Muscles of mastication- superficial group

3) **Medial pterygoid**: (Fig. 13)
    - O: lat pterygoid plate + maxilla
    - I: med side of angle of mandible
4) **Lateral pterygoid**: (Fig. 13)
    - O: Lat pterygoid plate + greater wing of sphenoid
    - I: condylar process of mandible

- **NS**: mandibular N (CN V3)
- **Action**: movement of the mandible in mastication

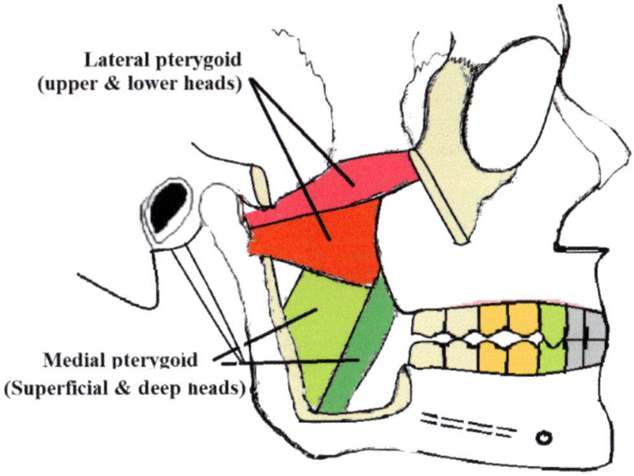

Figure 13: Muscles of mastication- deep group

<u>Deep muscles of the neck:</u> Muscles of Swallowing

Process of swallowing (Fig. 14)

1) The **tongue** and the **buccinators** push the **food** back opposite the roof of the mouth → passes to the pharynx (posterior throat).
2) **Suprahyoid muscles** → pull the **hyoid bone** upwards → **pulls the larynx upward**.
3) The **epiglottis** lies over the opening of the larynx → preventing food from entering the trachea.
4) *Levator palatini muscles* pull the **soft palate upwards →** preventing food from passing to the nose
5) **Pharyngeal constrictor muscles (superior, middle & inf)** push the **bolus** of food down the pharynx.
   - the inferior one overlaps the middle & upper ones
   - O: mandible + med pterygoid plate + hyoid bone
   - I: post raphe
   - NS: vagus (CN 10)
6) **infrahyoid muscles** return the hyoid bone and larynx to their original position.

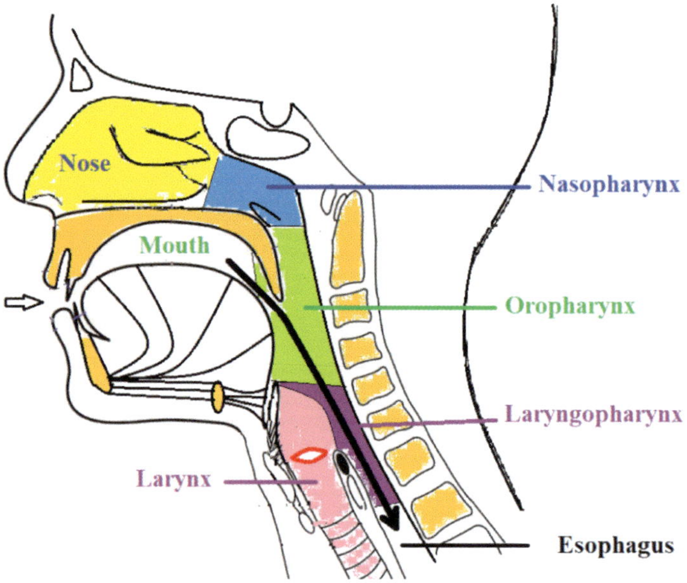

Figure 14: Pathway of food (swallowing)

Superficial muscles of the neck

They move the head (Fig 15)

1) **Sternomastoid**:
   - O: manubrium + medial clavicle
   - I: mastoid process + super nuchal line
   - NS: C2,3 + spinal accessory N (CN 11)
   - Action: turns head to opposite side
2) **Trapezius**:
   - O: occipital bone + lig nuchae + spines of C7 + all T
   - I: acromion + spine of scapula + lat 1/3 of clavicle
   - NS: spinal accessory N (CN 11)
   - Action: ext + add + med rotation of arm, help head extension

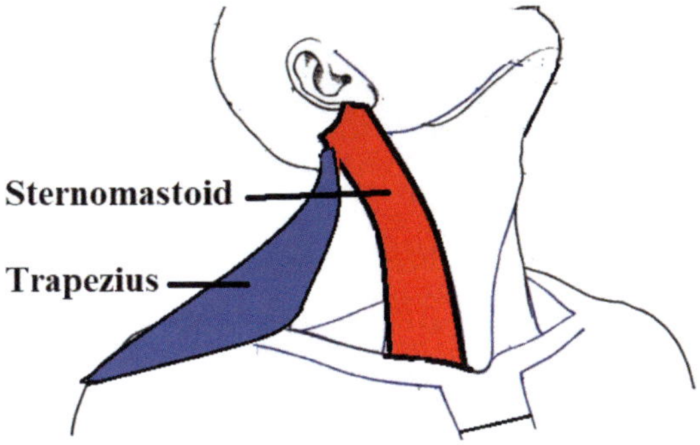

Figure 15: superficial muscles of the neck

Muscles of the trunk

<u>Muscles of the thoracic wall</u> (Fig 16)

External intercostal:

- Its fibers run **down & forwards**
- O: inf border of rib above
- I: upper border of rib below
- NS: intercostal Ns
- Action: pull the ribs up

Internal intercostal:

- Its fibers run **down & backwards**
- O & I: are the reverse of the above
- NS: intercostal Ns
- Action: pull ribs down

Diaphragm: dome shaped

- O: Xyphoid process + lower 6 CC + L1-3
- I: central tendon
- NS: phrenic N (C 3,4,5)
- action: the dome flattens in **inspiration**

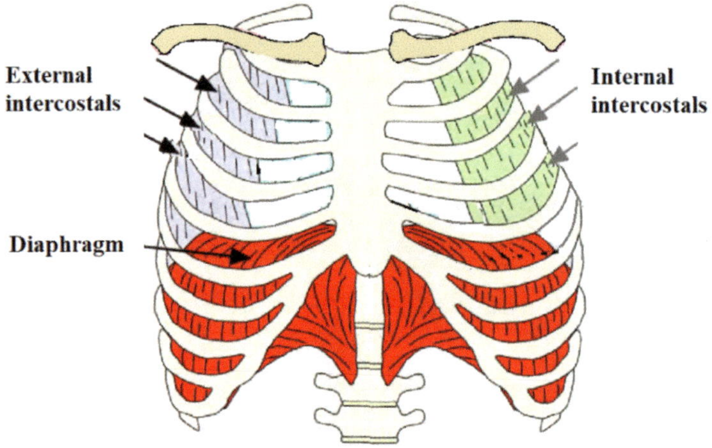

Figure 16: Muscles of the thoracic wall

<u>**Muscles of the abdominal wall**</u> (Fig 17)

Rectus abdominis

- O: pubic crest + symphysis pubis
- I: xiphoid process + costal cartilages 5,6,7

External oblique

- O: lower 8 ribs
- I: linea alba + pubic crest & tubercle + iliac crest
- Direction of fibers: down & med

Internal oblique

- O: lumbar fascia + iliac crest + inguinal lig.
- I: linea alba + pubic crest + last 3 ribs
- Direction of fibers: up & med

Transversus abdominis

- O: Ing. Lig. + iliac crest + lumbar fascia + last 6 CC
- I: linea alba + pubic crest
- Direction of fibers: horizontal

  - Action: Flex + rotate lumbar region
  - NS: intercostal Ns (T7- T12 + L1)
  - The transversus and oblique muscles of the right & left sides meet at the midline, forming the ***linea alba***

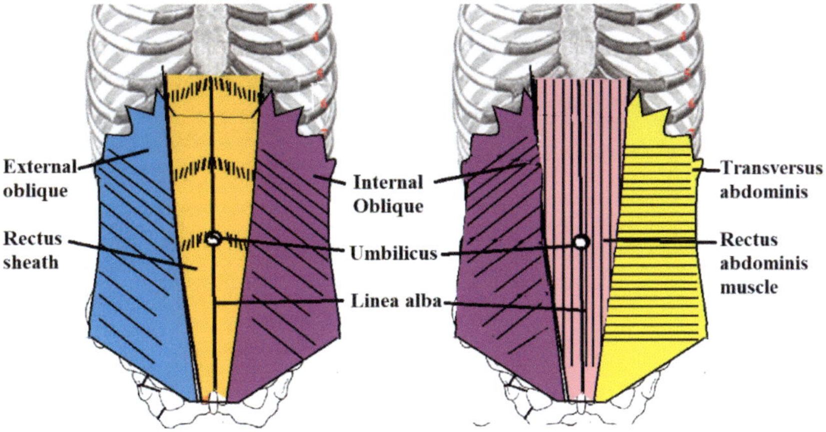

Figure 17: Muscles of the abdominal wall

Muscles of the Upper limb

Muscles of the shoulder

According to the **site**

- **Pectoral muscles**: in front of the shoulder region (Figs. 18, 19)
- **Scapular muscles**: on the back of the shoulder region (Fig. 20)

According to the **action**

- Muscles that **move the scapula:** attach the scapula to the thorax
- Muscles that **move the arm:** attach the scapula to the humerus

<u>Muscles that move the Scapula</u>

- **Trapezius** adducts the scapulae (Fig. 20).
- **Serratus anterior:** (Fig. 19)
  - holds the scapula in contact with the thorax
  - Pulls the scapula forward.
  - Causes a fast-forward movement of the arm → it is called the **boxer's muscle**.
  - Helps to **elevate the arm** above the horizontal level.

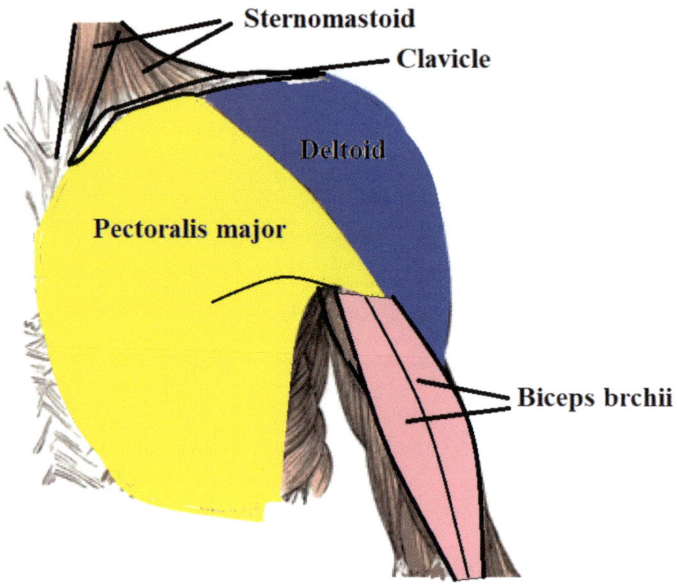

Figure 18: Pectoral region- Superficial muscles

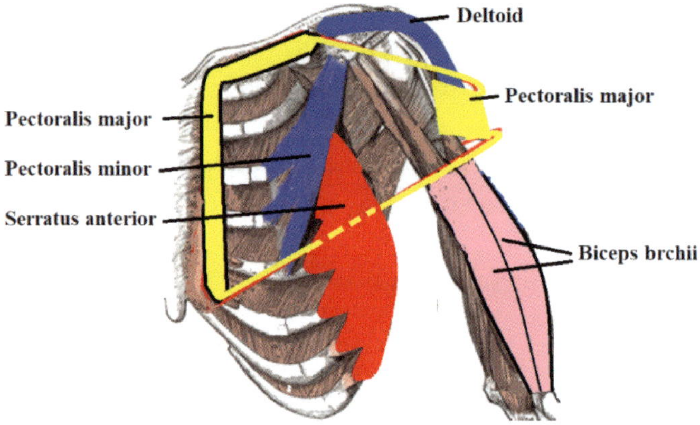

Figure 19: Pectoral region- deep group

<u>Muscles that move the Arm</u>

Deltoid: (Fig. 18)

- O: clavicle + acromion + spine of scapula
- I: tuberosity of humerus
- NS: axillary N
- Action: abd of arm

Pectoralis major: (Fig. 19)

- O: clavicle + sternum + CC 1-6
- I: intertubercular sulcus of humerus

- NS: med & lat pectoral NS
- action: flex, add & med rotation of the arm

Latissimus dorsi: (Fig. 20)

- O: lumbar fascia + lower T6 spines + L spines + lower 3 ribs
- I: floor of intertubercular sulcus of humerus
- NS: thoracodorsal N
- Action: ext, add & med rotation

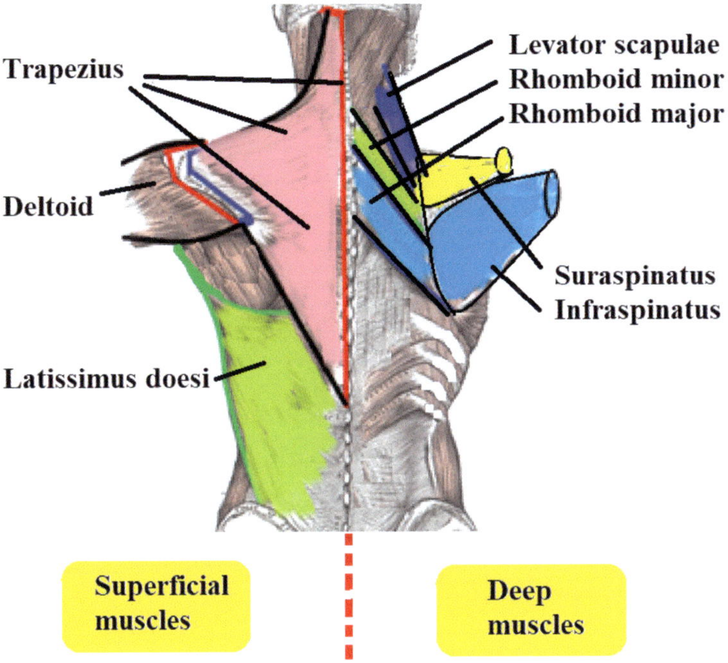

Figure 20: Superficial and deep muscles of the back

<u>Rotator cuff muscles</u> (Fig. 20)

- They lie deep to other muscles
- their tendons form a cuff around the shoulder joint
- **anterior to scapula**.
  - subscapularis muscle
- **superior to scapula**.
  - supraspinatus muscle
- **posterior to scapula**:
  - infraspinatus
  - teres minor

Muscles of the arm

Biceps (Fig. 21)

- O: coracoid process + supraglenoid tubercle
- I: radial tuberosity
- Action: flex & supinate forearm + flex the arm

Brachialis (Fig. 21)

- O: ant surface of humerus
- I: coronoid process of ulna
- Action: flex forearm
- NS: musculocutaneous N

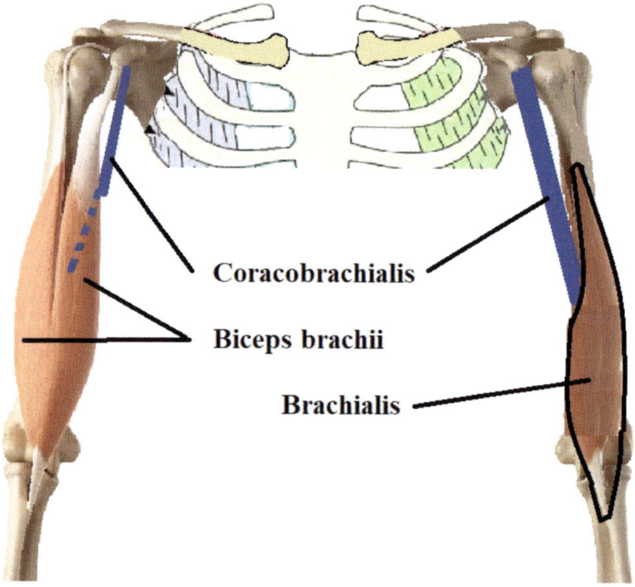

Figure 21: Muscles of the front of the arm

Triceps: (Fig. 22)

- O: infraglenoid tubercle of scapula (long head) + post shaft of humerus above (lat head) & below (med head) the spiral groove
- I: olecranon process of ulna
- Action: ext forearm
- NS: radial N

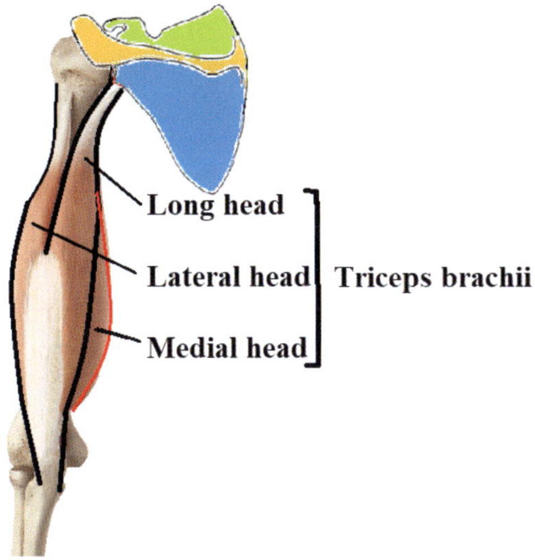

Figure 22: Muscles of the back of the arm

Muscles of the forearm

- They move the hand and fingers.

Flexors are on the anterior and medial forearm (Figs 23, 24)

- **flexors** flex the wrist and fingers

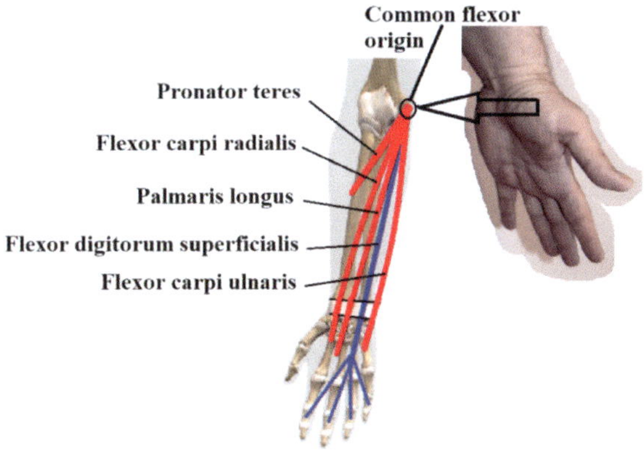

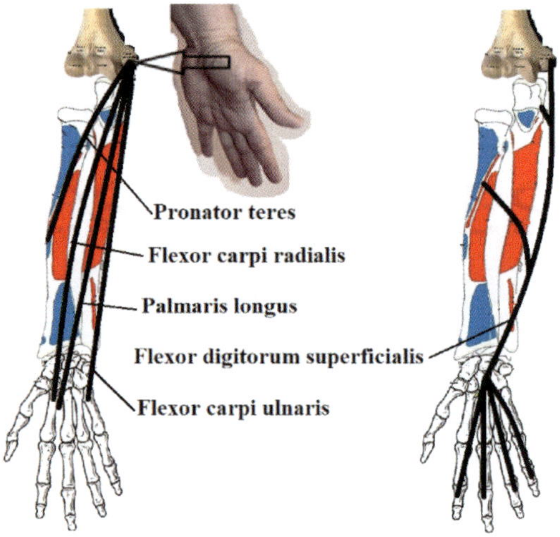

Figure 23: Superficial muscles of the front of the forearm

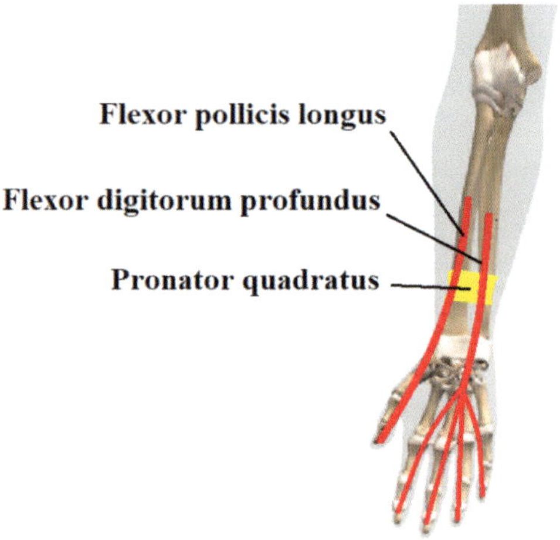

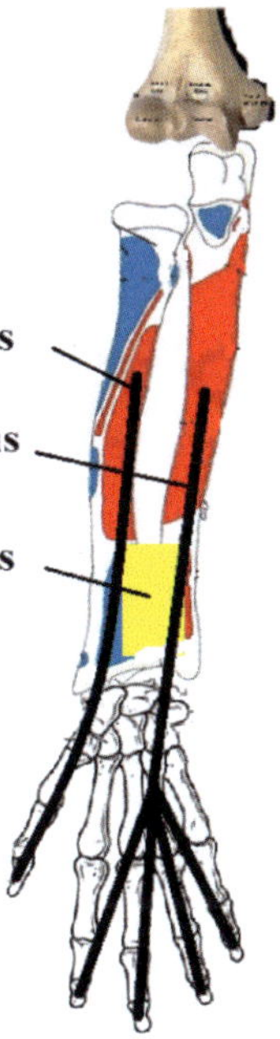

Figure 24: Deep flexors of the front of the forearm

<u>Extensors</u>: are on the posterior and lateral forearm (Figs 25, 26)

- **extensors** extend the wrist and fingers

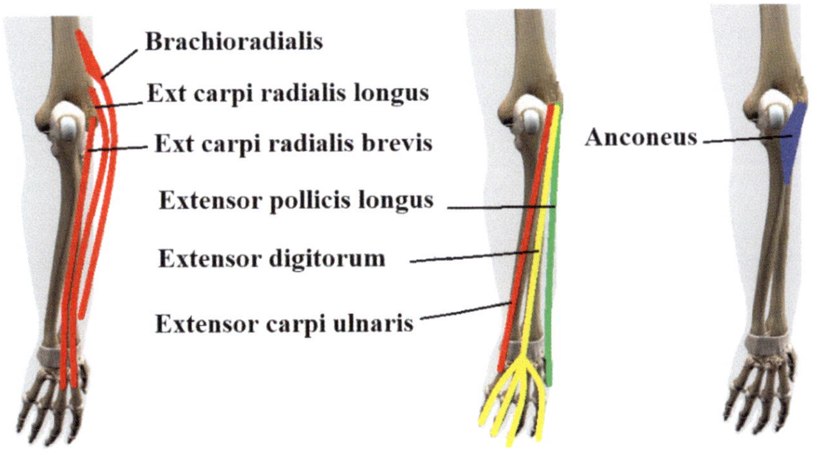

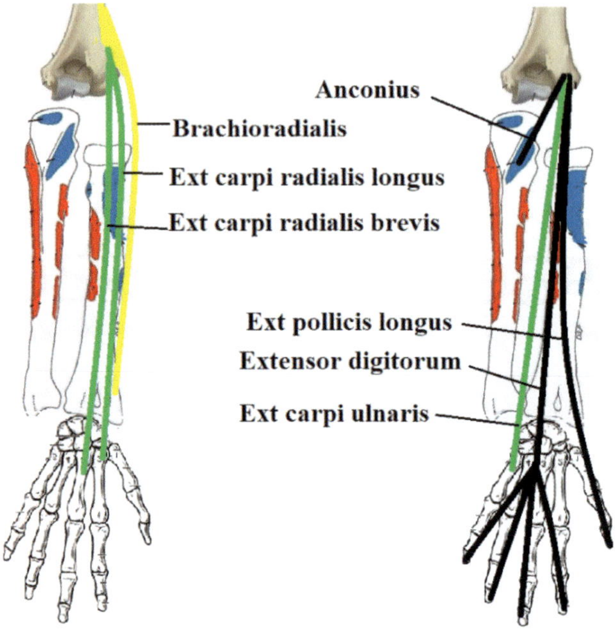

Figure 25: Extensor muscles of the forearm- superficial group

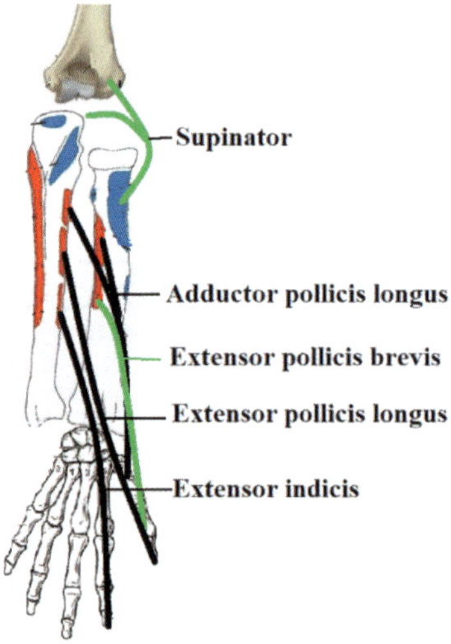

Figure 26: Extensor muscles of the forearm- deep group

- **Flexor carpi** and **extensor carpi** muscles
  - O: humerus
  - I: the bones of the hand.
- **Flexor digitorum** and **extensor digitorum** muscles
  - O: humerus
  - I: the bones of the hand.

Muscles of the Lower Limb

- They are large muscles because of their function
- Function:
  - to move the entire weight of the body
  - to resist the force of gravity.

Muscles that move the thigh

- O. the pelvic girdle
- I. the femur
- Movements of the **thigh** at the **hip joint**
  - thigh flexes, extends
  - thigh adducts, abducts
- Muscles of the thigh
  - **iliopsoas** lies anterior
  - **Gluteal muscles** lie posterior
  - **adductor** muscles lie medial

Iliopsoas (Fig. 27)

- includes psoas major + iliacus
- O: ilium and the bodies of the lumbar vertebrae
- I: on the medial femur
- Action
  - **flexing the thigh:** is the prime mover
  - Flexing the trunk (as in bowing)
  - is important in **walking & standing**

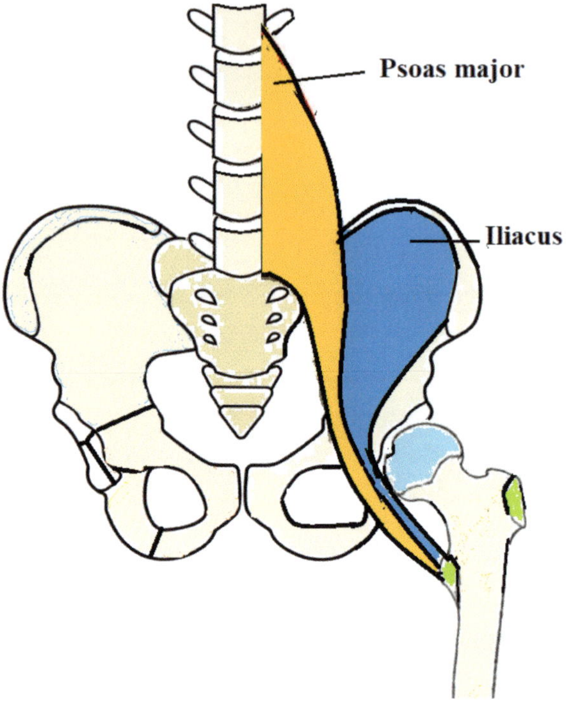

Figure 27: Flexor muscles of the thigh

Gluteus muscles

Gluteus maximus (Fig. 28)

- is the largest muscle in the body
- O: Dorsal surface of ilium + sacrum + coccyx
- I: Gluteal tuberosity of femur + iliotibial tract
- NS: inf gluteal N
- Action:
  - is the prime mover of thigh **extension**, Abd, lateral rotation
  - Is important in walking, climbing stairs, or jumping

Gluteus medius (Fig. 28)

- O: Lateral surface of ilium
- I: Greater trochanter of femur
- NS: sup gluteal N
- Action: **Abd, med rotation** of the thigh

Gluteus minimus (Fig. 28)

- Lies deep to the previous glutei

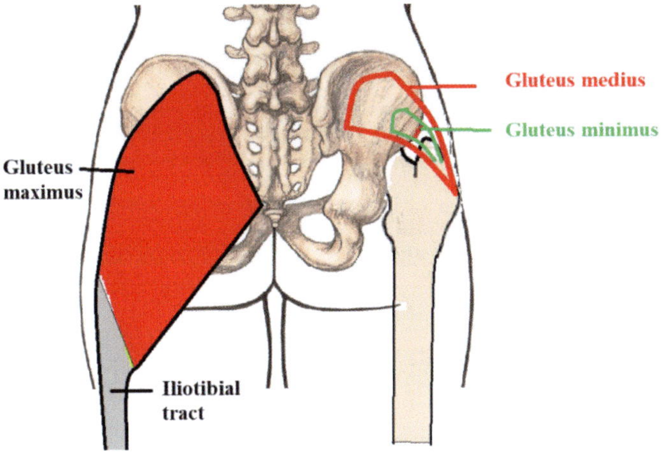

Figure 28: Gluteal muscles

<u>Adductor muscles</u> (Fig. 29)

- located on the medial thigh
- O: pubis and ischium
- I: femur
- Adductor muscles are
  - pectineus
  - adductor longus
  - adductor magnus
  - gracilis
- Action:
  - **adduct** the thigh
  - squeeze the thighs together (as in keeping a rider on a horse)

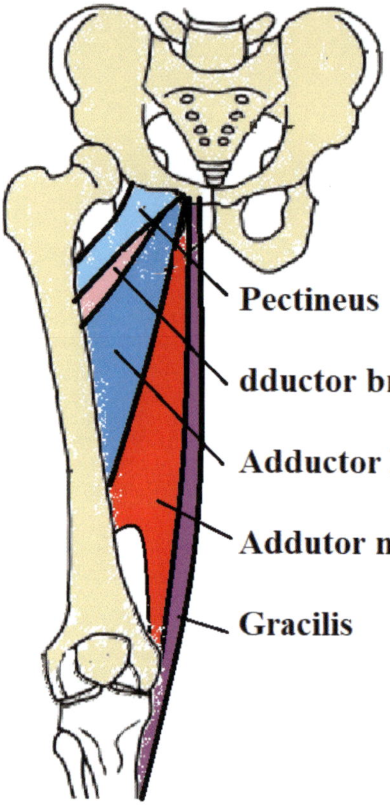

Figure 29: Adductor muscles of the thigh

Muscles that move the Leg

- O: from the pelvic girdle or femur
- I: on the tibia
- Muscles (Fig. 30): Sartorius, quadriceps femoris, hamstring

Sartorius: (Fig. 30)

- is a long muscle
- O: the iliac spine (ASIS)
- I: medial side of the upper tibia
- Action:
  - it acts on both the thigh & the leg.
  - **flexes both the leg and the thigh**.
  - **abducts and laterally rotates the thigh**, enabling us to **sit cross-legged**, as **tailors** used to sit in old times (*sartor* = tailor)

Quadriceps femoris: 4 muscles (Fig. 30)

- Rectus femoris
- vastus medialis
- vastus intermedius
- vastus lateralis

Rectus femoris:
- O: from the ilium
- I: patella + tibial tuberosity of ulna (through the patellar lig)

Action of quadriceps femoris:
- the primary **extensors of the leg** (as in kicking a ball)
- stabilize the hip
- assist in **thigh flexion**

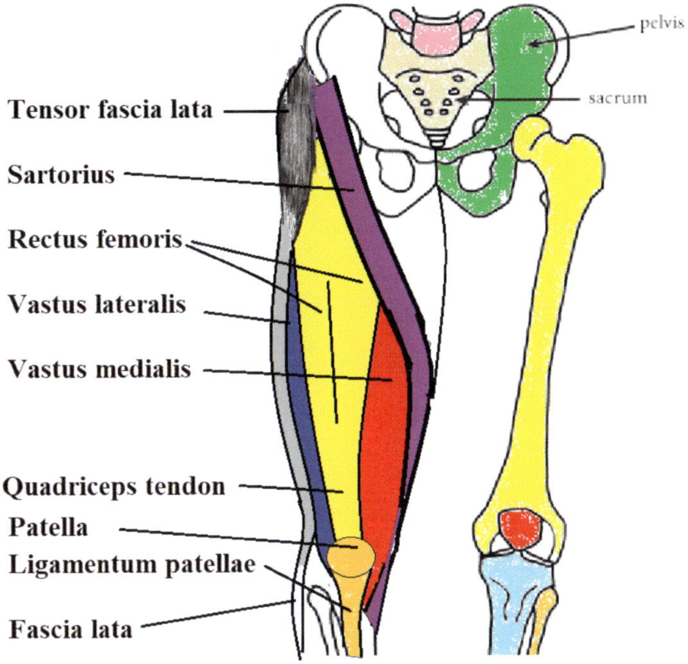

Figure 30: Front of the thigh

<u>**Hamstring muscles:**</u> 3 muscles (Fig. 31)
- Lat:
  - **Biceps femoris**
- Medially
  - **Semitendinosus**
  - **Semimembranosus**
- They cross the hip and knee joints
- O: ischium
- I: tibia.
- Action:

- **flex** and rotate the **leg** medially or laterally
- **extend the thigh**.

- Their tendons can be felt behind the knee
- They are used by butchers as **strings** to hang up **ham** for smoking

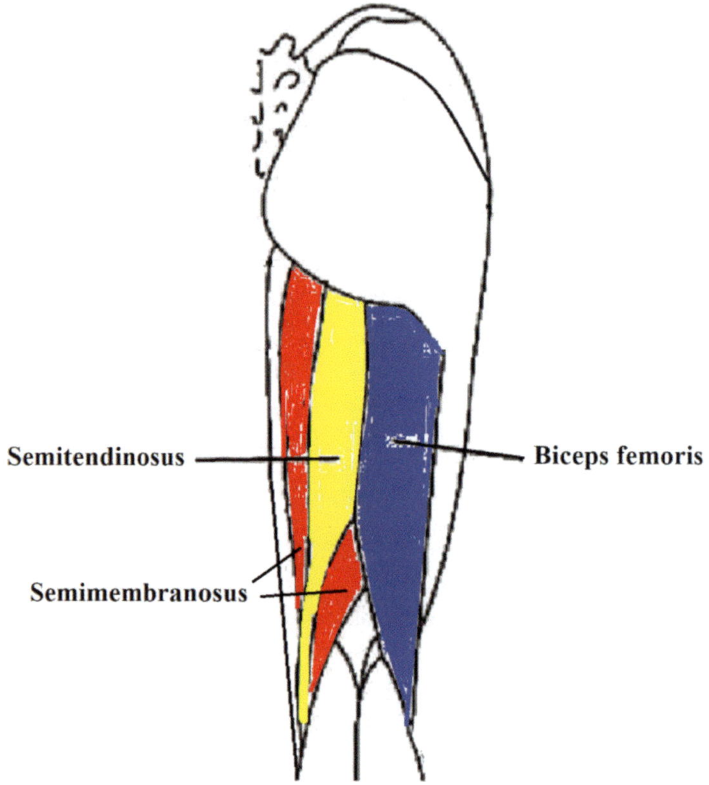

Figure 31: Hamstring muscles

Muscles That Move the Ankle and Foot

Gastrocnemius (Fig. 32)

- Site: posterior leg, forming the calf
- O: the femur
- I: joins the **calcaneal tendon** → which attaches to the calcaneus bone (heel)
- Action:
  - **leg flexor**
  - **plantar flexor of the foot** that aids in pushing the body forward during walking or running.
  - It is called the "**toe dancer's muscle**" because it allows a person to stand on tiptoe.

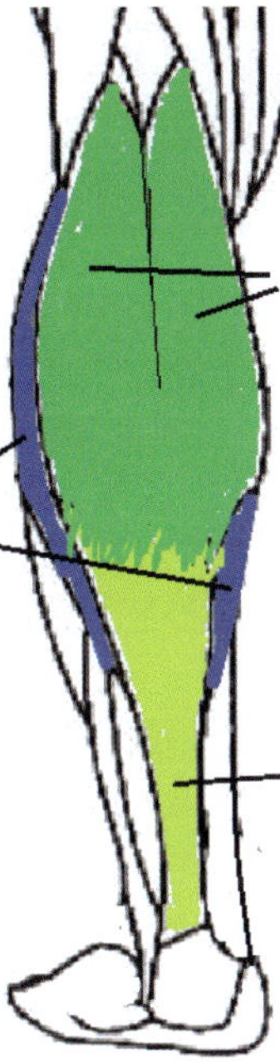

Figure 32: Muscles of the back of the leg

Tibialis anterior (Fig. 33)

- Site: at the anterior leg.
- O: ant surface of tibia
- I: the bones of the ankle and foot.
- Action: **dorsiflexion** and **inversion** of the foot.

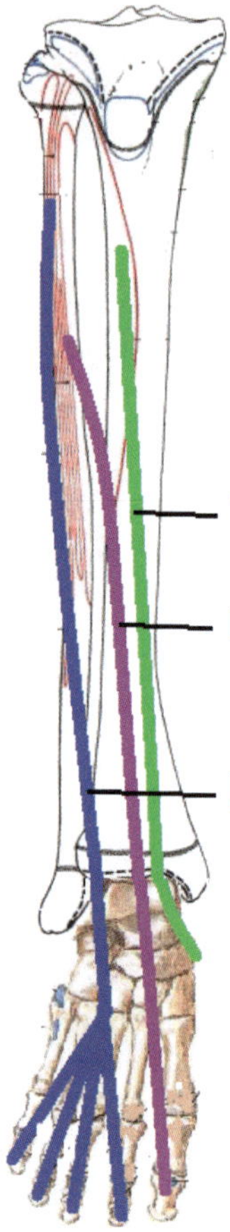

Figure 33: Extensors of the leg

Fibularis (peroneus) muscles (longus, brevis) (Fig. 34)

- are found on the lateral leg
- connecting the fibula to the metatarsal bones of the foot.
- Action:
  - **evert** the foot
  - help in **plantar flexion**.

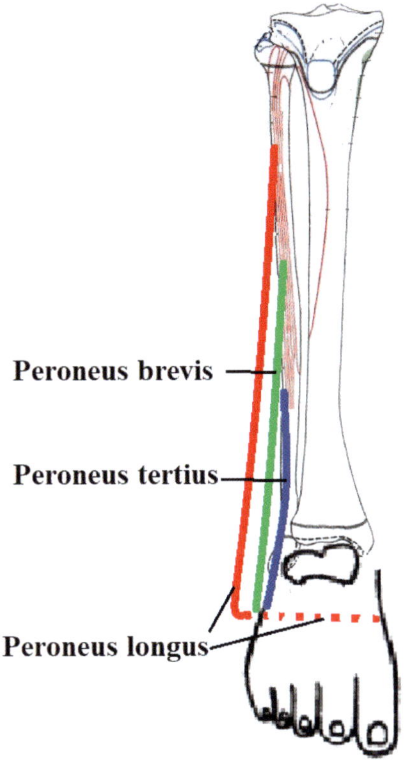

Figure 34: Lateral muscles of the leg

Flexor and extensor digitorum longus (Fig. 33)

- O: from the tibia
- I: on the toes.
- Action:
  - flex and extend the toes, respectively
  - assist in other movements of the foot

Effects of Aging and benefits of exercise

Effects of aging

- Lack of exercise and/or poor diet → decrease of **muscle mass** and **strength** → muscles are replaced by connective tissue → then fat.
- Degenerative changes in the **mitochondria** → endurance decrease

Benefits of exercise

- Builds up **muscles**
  - training **with weights** → improve muscular strength and endurance
- saves **skeleton**

  - training stimulates the activity of **osteoblasts** (bone-building cells)
- Control **weight** and keeps blood sugar in the normal range.
- Protects **heart**, blood vessels
  - Lower LDL
  - increases HDL
- Good for the **brain**
  - Prevent depression
- Helps to prevent **cancer.**

Appendix 1: learning objectives

Musculoskeletal system

1. Identify the major bones that make up the axial and appendicular skeleton and summarize their main differences.
2. Outline the main differences between compact and spongy bone.
3. Describe and contrast different types of joints (synovial, fibrous and cartilaginous) and their associated structures (cartilages, tendons, ligaments, and bursa) in relation to movement and stability.
4. Identify the microscopic structure of the skeletal muscle and the mechanism of performing its function.
5. Name and describe the major muscle groups of the head, neck, thorax, abdomen, pelvis, upper limb and lower limb.
6. Identify the main curvatures and features of the vertebral column, individual vertebrae (cervical, thoracic, lumbar, sacral and coccygeal) and intervertebral joints.

Appendix 2: Bibliography

1. Connolly et al.: Core anatomy syllabus for Undergraduate Nursing. Journal of Anatomy, 2018, 232: 721-728, published by John Wiley & Sons Ltd.
2. Elain Marieb and Katja Hoehn: Human Anatomy & Physiology, 11th edition. 2010, Pearson.
3. Lauralee Sherwood: Fundamentals of Human Physiology, 4th edition. 2011, Brooks/Cole, USA
4. Gerard J. Tortora And Bryan Derrickson: Principles of Anatomy and Physiology, 14th Edition, 2014 John Wiley and Sons, USA.
5. Memmler's the Human Body in Health in Disease Author: Cohen, Wood, and Memmler Publisher: Lippincott Williams & Wilkins Year: 2018 ISBN: 978-1496380500
6. Gray's Basic Anatomy, Richard Drake, Wayne Vogl, and Adam W. M.□, 2nd Edition, Elsevier Philadephia, 2017.
7. Mader S, Windelspecht M. Human Biology. 13th Edition. McGraw-Hill Science/Engineering/Math. 2013
8. Young B, Lowe J, Stevens A, Heath J, Deakin P. Wheater's Functional Histology: A Text and Colour Atlas. 6th Edition. Churchill Livingstone.2013.
9. John E. Hall. Guyton & Hall Text Book of Medical Physiology. 13th Edn. Elsevier Philadephia, 2016.
10. Koeppen, & Stanton. Berne & Levy Physiology. 7th Edition, Elsevier. 2018.
11. Barrett K, Barman S, Boitano S, Brooks H. Ganong's Review of Medical Physiology. 26th Edition. LANGE Basic Science. 2019
12. Human embryology Keith. L. Moore 5th edition.

Appendix 3: Human A&P Booklets

The following parts are available as **e-booklets**:

- Part 1/7: Introduction to A & P + Integumentary system
- Part 2/7: Skeletal and Muscular systems
- Part 3/7: Cardiovascular system and Blood
- Part 4/7: Respiratory and Immune systems
- Part 5/7: Digestive and Endocrine systems
- Part 6/7: Urinary and Reproductive systems
- Part 7/7: CNS & Special Senses

The 7 parts are compiled and published as a single **paper booklet** entitled: "**Human Anatomy & Physiology Booklet with Clinical Implications**"

Printed in Great Britain
by Amazon

62365765R00049